# CHILD ABUSE AND CULTURE

# CHILD ABUSE AND CULTURE

## Working with Diverse Families

### Lisa Aronson Fontes

*Foreword by Jon R. Conte*

**The Guilford Press**
New York   London

© 2005 The Guilford Press
A Division of Guilford Publications, Inc.
72 Spring Street, New York, NY 10012
www.guilford.com

Paperback edition 2008

Printed in the United States of America

This book is printed on acid-free paper.

Last digit is print number:   9   8   7   6   5   4   3

**Library of Congress Cataloging-in-Publication Data**

Fontes, Lisa Aronson.
  Child abuse and culture : working with diverse families / Lisa Aronson Fontes.
     p. cm.
  Includes bibliographical references and index.
  ISBN-10: 1-59385-130-8   ISBN-13: 978-1-59385-130-9 (hardcover)
  ISBN-10: 1-59385-643-1   ISBN-13: 978-1-59385-643-4 (paperback)
  1. Child abuse—Cross-cultural studies.   2. Interviewing in child abuse.   3. Child welfare workers.   I. Title.
  HV6626.5.F66 2005
  362.76′53—dc22
                                                          2004026524

*To my father, who always believed in me*

*And to my mother, my greatest cheerleader,*
*editor, and role model*

# About the Author

Lisa Aronson Fontes, PhD, is a Core Faculty Member in Union Institute & University's PsyD Program in Clinical Psychology. She has dedicated almost two decades to making the social service, mental health, criminal justice, and medical systems more responsive to culturally diverse people. Dr. Fontes edited *Sexual Abuse in Nine North American Cultures: Treatment and Prevention* (Sage, 1995), authored *Interviewing Clients across Cultures: A Practitioner's Guide* (Guilford, 2008), and has written numerous journal articles and chapters on cultural issues in child maltreatment and violence against women, cross-cultural research, and ethics. She has worked as a family, individual, and group psychotherapist, and has conducted research in Santiago, Chile, and with Puerto Ricans, African Americans, and European Americans in the United States.

Dr. Fontes earned a doctorate in Counseling Psychology from the University of Massachusetts and a master's degree from Columbia School of Journalism. In 2007 she was awarded a Fulbright Foundation Fellowship, which she completed in Buenos Aires, Argentina. Dr. Fontes is fluent in Spanish and Portuguese and is a popular conference speaker and workshop facilitator.

# Foreword

Our field of child abuse appears to be in the early stages of a great transformation. It is not completely clear which new ideas, models, data, and theories will contribute to this momentous change. It does seem increasingly clear that a significant aspect of this paradigm shift will be to leave behind the Eurocentric cultural blinders that have characterized our past practice, and to see the worlds of our clients for the multicultural rainbow they always have been.

This transformation began with an increasing understanding of the negative impact of white privilege, cultural imperialism, and racism. Unfortunately, for years the field has been stuck at this stage of sensitivity and has not been able to move toward a practice that embraces this understanding. Now a few of our colleagues have moved beyond sensitivity or consciousness raising to help us understand a new approach that is based on true multiculturalism, diversity, and cultural competence.

Lisa Fontes has produced a work of scholarship that must be seen as a major step toward achieving this transformation. It moves beyond calling attention to the problem to actually helping the field understand what multiculturalism and cultural competence mean in practice. This well-written book helps the reader develop a fuller awareness and appreciation of culture's impact on child abuse and on our work. Importantly, it does much more than that: It describes the skills and everyday actions that make up culturally competent practice.

This book contains numerous specific examples from a wide range of cultures that help us understand the many ways in which culture is relevant to child abuse intervention. These examples provide models for what to listen for in work with clients, and they sensitize the reader to the subtle ways in which culture may operate. I appreciate the author's willingness to make it clear that honoring diversity does not mean refraining from taking

any definite stance. Fontes takes such a stance herself in calling for an end
to all forms of violence against children, including spanking.

These days, the demand for "evidence-based practice" has become an
easy way to discount ideas that differ from one's own. Fontes has done an
excellent job of differentiating between research-based ideas and ideas
that arise from her own and others' expert practice. This is an evidence-
based book. However, to the author's credit, she has devoted considerable
intellectual and applied time to working out ideas for the rest of us. Fontes
clearly lets us know which concepts are based in research and which derive
from her own (and her colleagues') experience, and we are enriched by
reading the products of her thinking in both areas.

This is also a practical book with numerous specific suggestions about
how to perform assessments, interview children, work with interpreters,
and conduct many other aspects of multicultural child abuse practice. As
useful as these are, to me the greatest contribution of this book is the extent
to which it communicates a deep appreciation for and understanding of
the situation of children, adults, and families from diverse cultures who are
involved in the child welfare system. This empathic presentation draws the
reader into the discussion in an almost visceral way.

This book should become an indispensable part of the education and
continued training of social workers, psychotherapists, medical and legal
personnel, and law enforcement officers who work with diverse families
affected by child maltreatment. It has a great deal to offer beginning and
advanced practitioners alike. As we all become versed in its insights, we
will transform our field, and all families will receive the best possible
professional response to child maltreatment.

JON R. CONTE, PHD
*University of Washington*

# Preface and Acknowledgments

What does it mean to be "culturally competent" in child maltreatment work? It means we must be sincerely open to all forms of human diversity: ethnic culture, gender, social class, sexual orientation, ability, nationality, language, religion, and so on. We must accept this diversity with our minds and our hearts, and learn how to work competently to address people's diverse needs and circumstances. But how do we implement these grand abstract ideas? What does it really mean to welcome diversity and work competently with people from cultures that differ from our own? How can we handle the feelings of surprise and discomfort that often accompany new ways of thinking and behaving? What is required of us in terms of acquiring skills, questioning deeply held assumptions, and changing the way we view our work, our clients, and the systems that are in place (we hope) to serve them? A multicultural orientation requires us to learn far more than how to greet or talk to people from various cultures. It requires us to do more than learn scattered facts about diverse cultural groups. It requires us to do more than simply know and work to overcome our own biases and limitations—although all this is crucial. A true multicultural orientation requires us to adopt an open, appreciative attitude about the diversity of our clients' cultural practices, beliefs, mores, and expressions, and to implement policies and procedures that increase fairness for diverse peoples.

This book is grounded firmly in the practical concerns of people who work to prevent and intervene in situations of child maltreatment. It offers examples and tips from the real world of ethnically diverse families who face injustice in the child welfare system.

If you have picked up this book, I expect you will agree that professional training, good intentions, and empathy alone are not enough. We must understand the role of culture in the maltreatment of children and in our interventions, and adapt our work accordingly. When you finish reading this book, I hope you will have a good idea about how to carry out your everyday professional encounters in a culturally competent way.

One stylistic point: In this book I include a number of quotes from unnamed sources. In some instances, instead of identifying the person who made the statement, I provide demographic descriptors (e.g., "Puerto Rican psychotherapy client"). These quotes are taken from unpublished portions of research that I have conducted. The published documents are cited in the reference list under my name.

## IT TAKES A VILLAGE TO WRITE A BOOK

I feel so grateful to so many people, it's hard to know where to begin. I have come to believe that it takes a village and the wisdom of our intellectual ancestors to write a book. I have been blessed with tremendous personal and professional support over the years.

I would like to thank Carlos Fontes, who has been my caring companion for more than two decades. He survived and thrived after a difficult childhood, always modeling for me the skills of resilience. I would like to thank Ana Lua and Marlena, who work compassionately and passionately for social justice every day, and Gabriel, who brings sunshine to us all: my three children let me know my life has been worthwhile. You are the axis around which I spin the rest of my life. Carmina, Moisés, Alda, and Eric: I love you!

I would like to thank many people at Springfield College, including the members of the Psychology Department, Information and Technology Services, and the Faculty Development Committee. I would like to thank Christine Soverow, Sherika Hall, and Lisa Zephyr for doing much of the library research, and to offer a special thanks to Chris for reading and commenting on the entire manuscript in one weekend.

I would like to thank Terry Hendrix, who had confidence in my first book, which laid the foundation for my career. Terry and Gracia Alkema helped me understand the publishing business a little better and introduced me to Jim Nageotte of The Guilford Press, who has been supportive, responsive, and knowledgeable—what more could anyone ask from an editor? For their insightful comments, I would like to thank the four anonymous reviewers.

I have made wonderful friendships with brilliant people in the child abuse, education, and social justice fields over the years, many of whom contributed to this book by sharing ideas, reading chapters, supporting my professional development, or all of the above. I cannot thank you enough for all you give me and the world. So, in alphabetical order, I offer warm regards to Veronica Abney, Bill Ayers, Amber Black, Sandra Bloom, Bette Bottoms, Linda Bowen, Toni Cárdenas, Marc Chaffin, Pamela Choice, Larry Cohen and the Prevention Institute, Sharon Cooper, Deb Daro, Deb Davies, Elda Dawber, Linda Delano, Deanette Derezotes, Bernardine Dohrn, Katherine Eagleson, Sharry Erzinger, Kathleen Coulbourn Faller, Candice Feiring, Jeff Edelson, David Finkelhor, Raelene Freitag and the Children's Research Center, Rachel Hare-Mustin, Jason Irizarry, Walter Lambert, Kee MacFarlane, Sarah Maiter, Ron Moyer, Margarita O'Neill, Fred Piercy, Carole Plummer, Bob Reece, Janine Roberts, Murray Straus, and Joan Tabachnik and Stop It Now! Thanks especially to Jon Conte, who thought I had something worth saying in 1992, and who has been a friend and ally ever since. Since 1987, APSAC (American Professional Society on the Abuse of Children) has led the way to improved cultural competence and better services in all aspects of child maltreatment intervention. To all my APSAC colleagues, a warm hug.

My extended family community includes brilliant people who have shared their expertise for this book, as well as their love in my life, including Karen Anderson, Juan Carlos Arean, Eric Aronson, Ilia Cornier, Leticia Arteaga, Bert Fernández, Elizabeth Fernández-O'Brien, Joshua Garren, Kim Gerould, Magdalena Gomez, Roberto Irizarry, Fernando Leiva, and Eduardo Reyes. Jerry Fox, Betty Garren, Lo En Haw, Hattie Hobson, Nobuko Meaders, Pearl Putnam, and Ira Sharkey helped me build my center—which has enabled me to reach out.

My gratitude and admiration to the people affected by child maltreatment who have trusted me with their stories in research and psychotherapy. We strive to be worthy of your confidence.

There is an expression in Portuguese, "Desculpa qualquer coisa," which essentially means, "Forgive anything that comes up." In writing this book I have struggled with complex and controversial topics. I ask for understanding on the reader's part. I have done my best to "get it right," but you may feel at times that I have missed the mark, or left out important information. If that is the case, please let me know and let your voice be heard in the field.

# Contents

Percebem! A alma não tem cor. Ela é colorida. Ela é multicolor. (Understand! The soul doesn't have a color. The soul is colorful. It is multicolored.)
—ANDRÉ ABUJAMRA (1995), FROM A BRAZILIAN POPULAR SONG


If you want to help me with what happened to me as a kid, then you've got to know about my background, and my religion, and about how people treat me when they see the color of my skin or hear my accent. You've got to really understand where I'm coming from, or we're just wasting time.
—PUERTO RICAN PSYCHOTHERAPY CLIENT WHO EXPERIENCED INCEST AS A CHILD

# CHAPTER ONE

# Multicultural Orientation to Child Maltreatment Work

Julia González and her family walked into the children's advocacy center. The center was easy to find—it was in the neighborhood where they lived—and Julia was delighted to see that all the signs were written in both Spanish and English. The bilingual receptionist greeted them warmly and asked whether they'd rather fill out the intake forms in Spanish or English. Julia noticed a large sign on the wall, written in several languages, announcing that the center did not share information with federal immigration services.

The paperwork had room for her to note everyone who lived in her household, including her mother, her sister, and her sister's family. Julia's family had been referred to the center because a Sunday school teacher had been reported for sexually fondling Julia's daughter, Aíxa, and another child.

The interviewer greeted the González family in a friendly manner and invited them into a private room, where they were joined by a family advocate. The two professionals switched comfortably between Spanish and English. Julia and her family felt respected, valued, and heard. While the interviewer met alone with Aíxa in another room, the advocate thanked the parents for coming into the center and praised them for working so hard for their children's welfare. The advocate explained the interview process and what would follow in great detail, and allowed the family to ask questions. They discussed some of the ways the parents felt unable to protect their children in their new country, and how the parents had no way of knowing that the Sunday school teacher would prove dangerous. Ms. González was relieved to discover how supportive the advocate was, and was

1

pleased because she didn't seem to blame the parents in any way for what had happened. The advocate also gave Ms. González brochures, in Spanish, about a variety of local agencies that she thought could be helpful.

Although of course they would have rather not been involved in the child protection system at all, the González family felt empowered by the encounter. That night, they told the upstairs neighbor that she was wrong: these social workers were not "kid snatchers." They were very nice people who were working on behalf of families.

The above is a fictional account of the beginning of a culturally competent child maltreatment intervention. It refers to only a handful of the ideas that are developed at length and in depth throughout this book about how to work in a culturally competent way with diverse peoples on issues of child maltreatment.

## ORIENTING CONCEPTS

As we embark on this discussion of cultural competence in child abuse intervention, we need a common conceptual map and vocabulary to guide us. This chapter clarifies some of the terms and concepts that I use throughout the book. Some of these terms, such as "race," continue to spark a great deal of controversy. The ecosystemic framework I introduce in this chapter shapes the interventions I recommend throughout this book.

## ECOSYSTEMIC FRAMEWORK

People who are affected by child abuse are nestled in a variety of social (and material) domains that are highly interconnected and interactive (Fontes, 1993b). Bronfenbrenner (1979) describes these various levels in the ecological system as akin to Russian nesting dolls. I have adapted his model to highlight the importance of ethnic culture and the social service systems (see Figure 1.1). The most intimate circle is the individual child, consisting of the child's genetic makeup, individual experiences, and developmental level. The second circle is the child's home and family. The third circle I call "ethnic culture," but in some cases aspects of culture other than ethnicity—such as religion—will be more important. The fourth circle I call "proximal social systems." It includes the child's neighborhood, school, treatment providers, and peer group. I call the outermost circle "wider social systems." This circle includes state and national policies that impact on all the other systems.

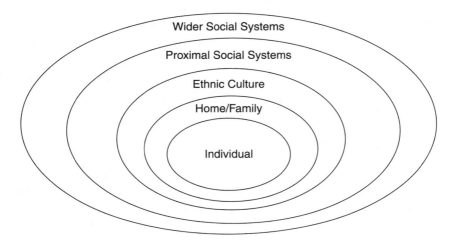

**FIGURE 1.1.** Ecosystemic framework for considering child maltreatment.

It is important to consider the various circles because they give us ideas for shaping our interventions. That is, we need to be widening and narrowing our focus constantly, like with a camera, to take into account all the aspects of the picture. If we focus in too narrowly, we may miss some of the contextual variables that would help us understand how to help a person—for instance, if we only conduct individual therapy with a child, we may overlook the way the child's poor achievement in school is affecting his self-concept; or if we interview one child only, we may neglect to intervene on behalf of his sister, who has also been victimized. On the other hand, if we widen our lens too broadly, we may miss some of the more proximal characteristics that are important to our work—for instance, if we offer a one-size-fits-all prevention program in a city, we may fail to notice that substantial numbers of families will not respond to that approach. Whatever our professions, our work will be improved if we widen and narrow our lens continuously, keeping in mind how our work influences and is influenced by the individual, his or her family, the ethnic culture, proximal social systems, and wider social systems.

This kind of model is not perfect. It artificially separates the different layers, which in reality influence each other mutually all the time (Rogoff, 2003). It is also unclear where to put forces like prejudice, which most likely impact a child through the proximal systems, and social problems such as poverty, that may result from a national policy but that can impact a child's life most intimately. That said, I think this model helps us in a number of ways:

1. It reminds us of all the various levels where we can intervene in a child's world. For instance, we can work with a child individually, with the child's family, with religious and cultural leaders, with the child's school and other treatment providers, and we can also try to improve municipal, state, and national policy. When our efforts are unsuccessful at one level (e.g., individual therapy), we can try widening or narrowing our focus to affect other systems.

2. It helps us move away from the overemphasis on the individual that characterizes Western cultures, inviting us to take into account family and community norms and concerns. This will put us more in step with clients who come from subcultures that value the family or the community more than the individual.

3. It helps us understand where we fit in the child's ecosystem. That is, if I am interviewing a child and I am not from that child's ethnic culture, I am one step further removed from that child. I will need to have some understanding of that child's ethnic culture before I can get close to him or her. On the other hand, I am also influenced and my work is constrained by forces larger than myself, including state and national policy, concerns about reimbursement, and so on.

## Ethnic Culture

"Culture is a set of beliefs, attitudes, values, and standards of behavior that are passed from one generation to the next" (Abney, 2002, p. 477). Culture defines what is natural and expected in a given group. We all participate in multiple cultures: ethnic, national, and professional, among others. We carry our cultures with us at all times, and they have an impact on how we view and relate to people from our own and other cultures.

Ethnic culture includes "language, worldview, dress, food, styles of communication, notions of wellness, healing techniques, childrearing patterns, and self-identity" (Abney, 2002, p. 477). Ethnic culture is what sets groups apart from each other, what gives them a sense of "us" and "them." Even after several generations live in North America, families retain traces of their countries of origin in their interaction patterns. That is, although after several generations in the United States a family that was originally from Sweden and one that was originally from Italy may look similar, if you closely examine their ways of relating within the family, their gender expectations, and their orientation to time, for instance, you will probably find traces of their countries of origin. Ethnic culture also affects the behaviors we consider abusive and nonabusive, a topic I discuss later in this book.

People from ethnic groups who look physically different from the American mainstream, often called "visible minorities," such as Japanese Americans, usually are made aware of their ethnicity frequently, as people may ask them where they are "from," no matter how many generations ago their family emigrated here. People from most White ethnic groups, on the other hand, are usually able to blend into the majority culture, and therefore may not harbor a strong sense of ethnic identity. After a couple of generations in North America many Whites feel like "regular" or "mainstream" Americans, a designation not frequently available to those from visible minority groups.

Ethnic cultures are not static. Rather, they evolve constantly as they come into contact with other cultures, are affected by history, and face the modernizing and homogenizing influences of globalization (e.g., television, movies, and the Internet). Entire cultures may shift dramatically over a relatively short period of time (witness the entrance of women into the workplace in Canada and United States in the last few decades and the striking social changes that have ensued). Individuals and families within ethnic cultures also change at differing rates, sometimes stirring up conflicts within families and ethnic communities.

Additionally, within a single family, members express their ethnic cultures to differing degrees and in different ways. For example, a Pakistani mother may wear traditional clothing, but buy takeout pizza for her family on her way home from work. Her husband may try to persuade their teenage children that their primary loyalty is not to their peer group but to their family, as is customary in Pakistan (Maiter, 2003), although he himself prefers watching televised baseball and basketball games over more traditional pursuits. Their teenage daughter may enjoy celebrating traditional religious holidays, but insist on having her navel pierced and getting a small tattoo on her back, like her multiethnic friends.

Ethnic cultures evolve as a whole. Moreover, there is also great variety within a given ethnic group (see the section below on stereotyping). We can never precisely describe an ethnic culture or community because they are multifaceted and change rapidly.

## Race

"Race" is a clumsy term. "Race" is commonly used to describe characteristics that appear to reside in the individual and to be biological in origin. People rely on physical markers such as skin color, hair texture, and the shape of the nose and eyes to identify membership in a group, and this group identity carries a great deal of social meaning. Clearly, however, the boundaries between the races are more social than biological. For instance, in the United States a person who is one-quarter African American (or Black) and three-quarters European American (or White) will typically identify and be identified by others as African American or Black, even if this person has light skin. The term "biracial" is only recently coming into more common use, but is still not a category used in the U.S. census. In Brazil, however, a variety of terms are commonly used to describe racial coloring, and someone with light skin but some African ancestry is not simply identified as "Black" or "White." Additionally, one's "race" clearly has a social meaning in North America that signifies relative power in the social system.

People who come from the dominant *racial* group, Whites, typically do not give a lot of thought to what it means to be White and the privileges that accrue from their skin color. McIntosh (1998) described this issue eloquently in her essay on Whiteness as being like an "invisible backpack" of privileges that White people carry around without awareness. Some of the privileges she mentions are knowing that one will not be discriminated against because of one's race when seeking housing or a bank loan; being able to go shopping without being followed or harassed; and routinely learning about one's history and culture in school, and having this be considered central to national history rather than meriting a month's "special" treatment. Nowadays, we should add to this list the freedom from police profiling and selective additional scrutiny by airport security forces. This is not meant to imply by any means that all Whites have a charmed life or don't suffer from other problems. Rather, it is just meant to acknowledge the advantages that accrue to Whites in the United States, Canada, and most of the world.

People who are not from the dominant racial group (non-Whites, or "people of color") are reminded daily of their race, but White people have the luxury of forgetting about their race. As a White Jew, I grew up acutely aware of my Jewish background and history, but I was literally unaware of the ways my White race benefited me. I am rather embarrassed to admit that I only began thinking about what it means to be White in graduate school, where I was flabbergasted to consider all I had formerly taken for granted.

I am increasingly convinced that it is important for White professionals to become aware of the privileges of their race. Only through this awareness can Whites truly begin to understand the experiences of non-White clients, who may be slow to trust people in positions of authority because of past negative experiences, and who may assume they will be mistreated, disregarded, or misunderstood by White professionals. It is important not to label these initial difficulties as simple "resistance," but rather to view them in their historical context. I believe it is also especially important for White people to speak out against racism and other forms of discrimination. People in the majority need to take on this struggle as their own and keep working to improve the general social climate.

## Professional Culture

We acquire professional culture through our training, reading, and daily interactions with colleagues. For example, a student I was supervising switched from using the word "teenagers" to using the word "juveniles" after just one day of shadowing a probation officer. Our socialization into professional culture often begins at colleges and universities, where typically there are small numbers of ethnic minority faculty and classmates to share their perspectives. Being educated and trained in such an environment contributes to a kind of professional ethnocentrism, where trainees from the dominant culture may come to see their worldviews and practices as being normal, and the perspectives of members of cultural minority groups as being aberrant or pathological, or at least "exotic." Members of ethnic minority groups who are trained in these institutions may also come to acquire these values.

Just as with our ethnic cultures, our professional cultures influence how we understand the world and the behaviors that seem normal, natural, and "right" to us. To put it simply, after years working in their own chosen fields, a law enforcement officer may come to see a family's actions in terms of what is legal and illegal, a psychoanalyst may come to focus on unconscious processes shaped by childhood influences, a social worker trained in systems theory is apt to look at the relationships between the family and their environment, an attorney may think about how parties involved would litigate the issues, and a physician is apt to focus on biological influences. Looking at the same family or "case," these professionals each bring along their own professional "lenses" and will view and describe the situation based on these perspectives. All these professionals will have to interrupt the tendency to jump to conclusions based on their training, and open their minds in order to truly understand each other and—more importantly—to understand the family's perspectives. The best we can hope for is to know our own backgrounds well and understand that our own view is but one way to see the world. If I am aware of my own biases I can avoid acting on them rashly.

When I meet with a family from a background that is different from my own, I bring all my professional and personal lenses with me. How I see the family is determined in part by how they compare with what I have known previously: people in my family of origin, other families with whom I've worked, and cases I have heard about. As much as I might like to, I am unable to view this family with lenses other than my own. This is why supervision by more experienced professionals, peer supervision, and teamwork are so important—other "eyes" on the case can enhance our own perspectives. Diverse treatment teams further improve our ability to see families from multiple perspectives.

## TREATING CLIENTS FAIRLY

In some sense this entire book can be seen as a plea and a plan to increase our ability to be *fair* to the diverse people we encounter in our work. Unfortunately, this is not as easy as simply "being a good person." Below, I describe some of the personal issues that impede our work. Elsewhere in this book I discuss these issues in greater depth, along with some of the structural barriers to fairness.

### Professional Ethnocentrism

Often professionals think about their clients' ethnic cultures but neglect to think about their own. This lack of attention to our own cultural upbringing increases the likelihood that we will act upon our assumptions as if they applied universally—we thereby practice ethnocentrism.

We do not stop being cultural beings when we become professionals. Rather, we layer our professional training onto our cultural selves. I heard a clear example of this recently when an Irish American physician told me the following story:

> "I think of myself as being relatively open-minded and unbiased. But while listening to your talk today I realized that I *do* respond differently to people of different ethnicities. For instance, if I am about to meet with an Italian or Latino patient, particularly a woman, I expect to encounter what we used to call in medical school, 'the mama mía syndrome'—that is, a *long* story about the history of the symptoms and a lot of unrelated information and complaints that could take up half my morning."

This agreeable and well-meaning physician said she therefore approached these Italian and Latina patients in a manner that discouraged them from divulging too much information—because she didn't have the time. Here we see the clashing of multiple cultures: the Italian or Latino valuing of context, stories, and connection versus the mainstream American medical culture of "Just the facts, ma'am," an attitude that has been aggravated by the time pressures of managed healthcare. As the more powerful individual in the encounter, the physician sets the tone. The patient is apt to pick up on the physician's impatience and therefore cut his or her story short—perhaps leaving out valuable information. Feeling undervalued by the physician, the patient might turn away from Western medicine and toward traditional ethnic healers, who are more apt to listen to the full story.

Because the media and schools reflect their same values and norms, people who are from the dominant groups (White, mainstream Christian, born in the United States or Canada, upper middle class, and heterosexual) are particularly likely to see the way they act as "normal" and to see others who act in different ways as strange, abnormal, or in need of intervention. It can be unsettling for people from the dominant group to reflect on their own cultural way as just one option rather than as the "natural" way (Rogoff, 2003). The dominant culture is so pervasive that it can be as taken for granted as the air we breathe. Therefore, it is especially incumbent on members of the dominant culture to be self-reflective and respectful when they work with people who may have a different set of values and beliefs.

## Bias

Most people are raised as part of a cultural group with a sense of "us" and "them." Part of that sense includes stereotypes about the child-rearing practices of people from other groups. We may believe that people from certain groups are more likely to abuse their children physically; or to abuse alcohol or drugs; or to be more negligent or less concerned with children's welfare.[1] These biases or prejudices become especially problematic when professionals are in positions of power over people from other groups, such as when they are conducting an investigation. These biases can lead to children in dangerous situations being underprotected because of a feeling that "those people always treat their children that way." Alternatively, stereotypes can lead to assumptions of child abuse where none exist because of lack of familiarity with the culture in question (see Chapter 3).

Biases against members of specific cultural groups can manifest in many ways, subtle and overt, and have a tremendous cumulative impact. Bias can enter at all points, from the first suspicion of abuse to investigation to legal action. Bias can be present in the protective, criminal justice, legal, medical, and therapeutic spheres. Bias can result in negative outcomes ranging from failure to substantiate legitimate claims of abuse, which leaves children in danger, to falsely "substantiating" abuse, which removes children from homes unnecessarily. Biases contribute to the current situation in which White maltreating families involved in the child protective system are more likely to be referred to therapy and other supportive services, whereas racial and ethnic minority parents are more likely to face adversarial interventions (Tjaden & Thoennes, 1992).

Bias can stem from genuine dislike by providers toward members of certain groups, or well-meaning but equally destructive misunderstand-

---

[1] Black and White women use illicit drugs to the same extent, for instance, but Black women are 10 times more likely than White women to be reported for substance abuse during pregnancy (Azzi-Lessing & Olsen, 1996), reflecting a bias in reporting.

ings. Such bias can be illegal, legal, or even legally required, as in cases where children are removed from homes because of the sexual orientation of a parent involved in a custody battle, as happens in certain jurisdictions.

Biases can make us jump to the assumption that certain conditions are evidence of child abuse when a more careful assessment would reveal a medical or other cause. For instance, often children with Asperger syndrome refuse to make eye contact, retreat from touch, and demonstrate impaired interpersonal relations that could be interpreted as evidence of child abuse by someone unfamiliar with the condition. Another example: one common feature of sickle-cell anemia (a medical condition that is more common among people of African, Mediterranean, and southwest Asian descent than among other groups) is hand and foot syndrome, which is characterized by swollen hands and feet and accompanied by local pain that makes a child cry (Qureshi, 1989). Ringworm, a skin condition that causes circular scarring on a child's skin, may also be mistaken for cigarette burns. With each of these medical conditions, a professional who carries biases against members of a specific group might rush to suspect child abuse when spotting the above symptoms in children from that group. (See Chapter 3 for more examples of bias in assessments.)

Bias can also alienate children from their caretakers outside of their homes. For instance, when schools are overcrowded and underfunded, with inadequate staffing and leaky roofs, children may come to believe that they are not valuable. In these circumstances, children may feel they have nowhere to turn for help. An adult Puerto Rican woman who grew up in the United States and had been sexually abused by her uncle described her isolation at school: "There's so much emphasis put on the White people. I think they would have listened and done something if I was White." She had tried to disclose several times and had the impression that no one cared about her because of her ethnicity. In this case, the child was left at risk because of bias.

Members of minority groups, immigrant groups, economically oppressed groups, and gay men and lesbians often actively fear child protective agencies. These agencies are perceived as "child snatchers" who are eager to destroy their families (Armstrong, 1995). These fears have some basis in fact. Prejudice, lack of cultural understanding, and police brutality are realities in many communities. Racial and ethnic disproportionality in the child protection system is widely decried (this topic is discussed further, below). Black children, in particular, are at high risk for extended out-of-home placement, years in the foster care system, and permanent removal from their families (Charlow, 2001–2002; Roberts, 2002). If we child maltreatment professionals wish to gain the trust of poor and minority communities, we must earn it.

# Confronting Stereotypes

Stereotyping is using simple, general labels about a group of people to draw unwarranted conclusions about individuals from that group. We acquire stereotypes as we grow up and listen to the ways adults in our families and schools discuss people from various groups. Television and other forms of mass media also convey stereotypes.

As professionals, we may also acquire stereotypes through readings or training sessions that emphasize a "cultural literacy" approach to working with diverse people, an approach that provides information about members of specific cultures. Culture-specific information on working with people from particular groups can be quite helpful (see, e.g., Boyd-Franklin, 2003; Falicov, 1998; Fontes, 1995a; McGoldrick, Giordano, & Pearce, 1996). However, while information about specific cultures alerts us to some of the unique issues that may be important for people from that group and can help us design interventions, we should never use the information as stereotypes or recipes for how to work.

Only the clients can tell us how important a certain part of their identity is at any given point in time. For instance, for a young Black girl, Shewana, raised in a home with four older siblings, her position as "the baby of the family" may be most important until she attends school. When she attends elementary school, gender may become her primary identifier, as she is likely to choose other girls to play with and to engage with them in "girl" activities. Then, when she is 12, particularly if Shewana attends an interracial middle school, her race may seem to be a more important part of who she is and may be the first thing she thinks of when asked "Who are you?" If Shewana becomes an avid member of the spelling or basketball team, these identities may take precedence over the others. And if in high school Shewana converts to a new religion, her religious identity may become more salient for her. If a professional who meets Shewana thinks "Black child" and clicks into stereotypical thinking based on this categorization, the professional will miss seeing Shewana in all her distinctive individual glory.

Culture is complex and multifaceted. People who seem to be from the same culture may differ widely. Just knowing that John is a Chinese American, for instance, tells us little about how he lives. Does he speak Chinese? How many generations has his family been here? In what ways do he and his family accept and reject Chinese culture and the dominant U.S. culture? If he goes to a school with many Latin Americans, he may have adopted aspects of Latino cultures. Knowing that he is Chinese American is just the beginning of what we need to know about John to understand him culturally.

Saba and Rodgers (1990) write eloquently about the danger of stereotypical assumptions: "When we enter a situation believing we already know the answer, we close ourselves off to the possibility that perhaps we really do not know at all" (p. 187). As we work in the field over time, and as one family begins to remind us of another with whom we have previously worked, it is important to remain open to being surprised and to allowing each family to teach us about its own unique reality. I have heard professionals say that they "knew everything about the case" merely by reading the referral sheet or walking through the doorway of a family's home. It is important to guard against this overconfidence—a kind of stereotyping. Rather, as we begin working on a new case and have the privilege of meeting with a new family, it may be helpful to hold an attitude of "I wonder what I will learn by working with this family." This kind of open approach helps us guard against stereotyping.

Falicov (1995) recommends that we adopt an inquisitive and open-minded strategy rather than relying on stereotypical information about members of a particular group. She also cautions us to view people in all their many contexts and facets including "rural, urban, or suburban setting; language, age, gender cohort, family configuration, race, ethnicity, nationality, socioeconomic status, employment, education, occupation, sexual orientation, political ideology; migration and state of acculturation" (p. 375). In other words, knowing one particular fact about a family's identity, such as its race or ethnic background, tells us little about who the family really is.

Saba and Rodgers (1990, p. 205) offer the following guidelines:

1. Clarify your assumptions [about the members of the group];
2. Realize that your perceptions may vary considerably from the family's;
3. Accept that a climate of mistrust exists;
4. Understand that mutual stereotypes enter the interview room first;
5. Be conscious of the power relationships between you and the family;
6. When uncommon events occur, consider alternate explanations in addition to the obvious ones;
7. Accept and admit your fallibility;
8. When you discover your discriminatory behaviors, do not give up. Make changes and continue to work;
9. Explore your setting for structures that foster prejudice;
10. Cultivate safe collegial relationships which will permit discussion of clinical discrimination; and
11. Most importantly, be open to learning from the families you treat.

It is hard to confront our stereotypes. When we are called to task for acting in a discriminatory manner or telling an offensive joke, it is easiest to respond to the person who has pointed out the problem with some version of: "It was only a joke. . . . I didn't mean it the way you think. . . . You are reading too much into it. . . . You [people] are too sensitive." It is much harder to thank the person for taking the risk of confronting us, tell him or her we'll think about it, and then truly look into our hearts and actions to identify their source and their impact. If a joke is made without malicious intent but is offensive to the listener, it is probably not wise to make that kind of joke again. It is important to err on the side of compassion and civility.

Every year I teach a graduate class in counseling diverse populations in which adults of all ages are asked to examine the stereotypical thinking they were raised with concerning social groups (e.g., "What ideas did you learn in your family about White people?; What ideas did you learn in your family about poor people?; What ideas did you learn in your family about gay men?"; etc.). The students are asked to discuss how they learned these ideas, which of them they wish to retain, and which they wish to abandon. Most students find this to be a challenging and emotionally laden exercise. Although rarely do students remember being given lectures on "What people from X group are like," upon reflection they discover that their family members, teachers, and neighbors communicated stereotypes through what they said, did, and didn't do. Many students also describe being caught in a loyalty bind: if they are willing to admit to family prejudices and decide to discard them, they feel disloyal to their families.

Although confronting and abandoning stereotypes is a difficult process, I consider it one of life's greatest joys. Holding stereotypical views and acting in a discriminatory manner take their toll on the mental and physical health of *both* the target and the agent of prejudice (Bowser & Hunt, 1996). Abandoning our prejudices and stereotypes is like cleaning and focusing our lenses. We experience the joy of knowing people as they truly are.

## From My Own Ethnic Group

I have heard professionals from various ethnic groups indicate that there are special challenges when working with client families who are from their own ethnic group, whether that ethnic group is from the majority or from a minority culture. Some of the challenges in child maltreatment work include:

• A temptation to deny, minimize, or overlook abuse because it is too hard to admit publicly that people who are "like me" have hurt or neglected their children. We may want to protect these "similar" individuals from getting caught up in the child welfare and criminal justice systems. We may also hesitate to admit to our colleagues that these people—who may feel like extended family—have done wrong. We may find ourselves empathizing so strongly with the difficult situation in which parents find themselves that we overlook the harm that may befall their children.

•  A temptation to deny, minimize, or overlook abuse because it is too painful to admit to oneself that these children—who look like our own nieces and nephews—have been hurt.

•  Occasional difficulty obtaining complete information, as family members may say "You know how it is" and decline to elaborate, assuming that a racial or ethnic similarity gives the professional automatic insight and obviates the need for elaboration.

•  A temptation to accept what the parents say "at face value" in a way that we wouldn't do for members of another group. Caretakers of all groups may try to take advantage of this. A father from Puerto Rico may say to a social worker who is also Puerto Rican, "'*Mano* [brother], give me a break here. We *potorros* [Puerto Ricans] have to stick together." Similarly, a White upper-middle-class mother might use her self-assurance and a sense of entitlement to try to convey to a White social worker that *she*, unlike some of *those* parents, can address a problem by herself or with the help of a private therapist or physician, and *she* is not the kind of mother who needs the state poking into her business.

•  Difficulty speaking about sexual or other sensitive issues with members of one's own group because it is like insulting one's own family to bring up certain topics or to use forbidden words. (I have also heard people claim the opposite: that it is easier for them to discuss difficult topics with members of their own group.)

•  A temptation for professionals to judge more harshly someone from their same minority group. Professionals who have overcome poverty, racism, and other obstacles themselves sometimes dismiss as a "sob story" the explanations of families from a similar background. An attitude of "I made it, why can't you?" may surface.

In child maltreatment, issues of social class may supersede ethnic issues. That is, a middle-class African American professional who has been trained in the professional values of the dominant culture may not be perceived by a Black client as being similar at all. Smith (2002), an African American professor of psycho- and sociolinguistics who originally came from a low-income family, writes of his early mistrust of African American professionals: "I developed an intense mistrust and dislike for professionals, especially 'boozje' [bourgeois] Blacks. . . . Because Black professionals were always 'talking proper' and seemingly 'puttin' on airs,' they appeared superficial, insincere, and phony" (p. 19).

It is important for us to be aware of cultural issues, even when working with clients who are from our own ethnic culture. Additionally, supervisors should not assume that ethnic matching guarantees easy empathy—

for example, by believing that Latino professionals have an automatic "in" with Latino clients. Rather, an agency climate should be created in which each professional can speak openly about complications in working with clients for all kinds of reasons, including ethnic similarity or difference.

## Help Seeking

When our clients don't want the "help" we sincerely try to provide, it can baffle us, frustrate us, or even make us angry. Let's examine culturally varied views of help seeking. In workshops, I sometimes ask participants who their families turned to when facing a crisis while they were growing up. The results usually look something like this: African American participants say they turned to clergy or a senior member of the extended family; Latinos say they turned to a godparent or grandparent, to clergy, or directly to God; White Anglo-Saxon Protestants often say they had no crises growing up, but if they admit to such crises they say they could not imagine their parents turning to anyone outside the family; Jewish participants say their families would turn to a doctor or a psychotherapist; Irish participants say their parents would turn to a priest or a police officer; Cambodian participants say they turned to a monk or community elder; and so on. Clearly, ethnic culture can influence help-seeking strategies. What does this mean for us in terms of child maltreatment interventions?

First, some clients will be more comfortable than others, from the outset, with the idea of meeting with social workers, police, attorneys, psychologists, and medical professionals. People who are less familiar with our roles may need extra help in understanding them and trusting us.

Second, for some clients a referral to psychotherapy is a relatively straightforward matter; but for others this is the equivalent of saying they are "crazy." In general, I recommend using the word "counseling" instead of the word "therapy" with most families, and introducing counseling as "a way to learn some strategies that have been helpful to other people when coping with a stressful situation like yours."

Third, if we know families are turning to a variety of people for help, then we must think about how these other people are affecting our work, and find ways to involve them, where feasible. For instance, if a Cuban mother practices the Afro-Caribbean religion of *santería* and her child falls ill, she may consult her *santero* godparent before agreeing to comply with medical treatment (Martínez, 2003). And if this person suggests that what her child really needs is an initiation into the *santería* religion, either instead of or before the medical intervention, there is a good chance the mother will devote her energy and resources to the initiation ceremony and not to the medical intervention. To increase the likelihood of the mother's cooperation, the professional coordinating the child's care may need to get in touch with the *santero* and seek his or her help or support. The same would be true for clergy, extended family members, faith healers, practitioners of traditional medicine, and others. If the family is relying on these individuals and we can find ways to bring them onto our side, we can usually be more effective.

And finally, it is easy to grow impatient with caretakers who have not followed our recommendations and who appear to be "doing nothing" although their child is suffering. It is important to ask the caretakers what they *have* been doing—they may be engaged in an elaborate process to help a child recover that is invisible to us because it does not conform to the usual practices of our own culture.

## Considering Issues of Language

For clients who are unaccustomed to speaking Standard English, encounters related to child maltreatment intervention have an extra layer of tension. Imagine how hard it is for a child or adult who is accustomed to speaking African American Vernacular English (formerly called Black English) or Spanish or any other language who is approached by an authority around a threatening topic and expected to respond in a language that is not the language of his or her heart. Trinidadian scholar Joanne Kilgour Dowdy (2002) writes about the difficulty of having to speak in the "master discourse" rather than in "the language of personal expression" (p. 4):

> At a loss for words really describes the feeling of the soul in the "white" language world. Thoughts come into her head in her family's intimate vocabulary, and she strains to translate those ideas into the accepted form expected in public conversation. She expects that her usual facility with language will be available to her when she begins to speak in public. Instead, there are cold, metal sounds bouncing off her teeth, the act of translation cooling the passion of the thought. . . . The continual disappointment with the master discourse creates a shroud that covers every utterance with a doubt about its worthiness. The voice in her head does not match the tone in her throat. She sees and hears herself becoming a tape played at the wrong speed. (p. 12)

Our work with people around issues of child maltreatment should not be like this. With an open and warm attitude, we should convey that however they speak is just fine—we will listen, and we will do our best to understand.

If our clients do not speak English fluently, we should call in a qualified interpreter immediately (see Chapters 2 and 7). However, we still frequently need to converse with people who are not native speakers of English, or who may speak a form of English that is not familiar to us.[2] In these encounters we must be supportive and understanding, and we must make a concerted effort to understand the clients' speech without shaming them.

Small rejections of their language hinder our ability to set up a trusting relationship with people from a different cultural group. Delpit (2002) describes this eloquently: "Since language is one of the most intimate expressions of identity, indeed, 'the skin that we speak,' then to reject a person's language can only feel as if we are rejecting him" (p. 47). We must be careful, then, not to correct our clients' English, and not to show impatience if we are having trouble understanding them. Our responses to people who use different dialects of English are more than just responses to "difference"; they are responses to foreignness or poverty. Purcell-Gates (2002) asserts that "the language one speaks is the clearest and most stable marker of class membership" (p. 133). She continues:

> [The] dialects of those in power do not elicit the same knee-jerk disdain and assumptions of deficit as do the dialects of the sociopolitically marginalized. For example, the Boston dialect of the Kennedys or the Southern dialect of Jimmy Carter are never pointed to as evidence of cognitive and linguistic deficit. But let a poor, urban, Appalachian woman speak for only a few minutes and powerful attitudes of prejudice and assumptions of inferiority are elicited. (pp. 133–134)

Some professionals will hear people's speech and—on a gut level—assume that the way they talk marks them as stupid. This can be as true for White people who might be considered "hillbillies" or "White trash" as for immigrants and members of racial minority groups. We must guard against these responses, and know they are ingrained stereotypes based on perceptions of social class and difference.

## POVERTY

Looking at child abuse ecosystemically requires that we consider all the systems in which children are embedded, including their families, their neighborhoods, their peers, their ethnic and religious communities, and the wider society (Belsky, 1980; Fontes, 1993b). Each of these levels can affect a given family in such a way that maltreatment is more or less likely to occur. Access to economic resources can serve as a buffer to child maltreatment. For instance, in a safe neighborhood with adequate recreational facilities, children can keep themselves occupied, let off steam, and stay "out of the way"

[2]How many people from Canada and the United States realize that in England, the word "fanny" refers to a woman's pubic area as well as a person's backside?

of an irritable parent with a short fuse who may be unemployed and at home. (Of course, while these conditions are helpful, they do not guarantee the safety of wealthier children!)

On the other hand, in unsafe neighborhoods children often are kept inside in cramped quarters, increasing the likelihood of disciplinary encounters and the possibility that these will escalate into violence. If children from unsafe neighborhoods are permitted to play outside their apartments, they are more likely to be subjected to the dangers of the streets. One study noted a 21.7% prevalence rate of posttraumatic stress disorder (PTSD) among 7- to 18-year-old inner-city Black children (Fitzpatrick & Boldizar, 1993). Fully 70% of this population had been victims of violence, and over 40% had witnessed a murder. These levels of violence are almost unimaginable to most people. It is hard to fathom how anyone keeps children safe in these circumstances. This reality was driven home to me personally when, several summers ago, a 12-year-old girl from Harlem, Sherri, stayed with my family for 2 weeks, through a Fresh Air Fund program. As part of a departing gift, we gave her a soccer shirt from the local team. She tearfully declined it because the shirt was red. If she were seen wearing red, the color of the Bloods, a powerful gang, she could be targeted by members of a rival gang, the Crips. Even the color of her clothing could put her at risk, a danger that my own family had never faced, and never previously considered. "Everything is a crapshoot when you're poor," writes the poet Magdalena Gomez (2004), reminding us how hard it is for low-income parents to keep their children safe, healthy, and educated when there is so little support from wider social systems.

Child neglect is mainly concentrated in the lowest socioeconomic groups (Charlow, 2001–2002). When caretakers have fewer resources, it is simply harder to provide children with what they need; there is less margin for error. One stolen paycheck, one car accident, one sick but uninsured family member, and an entire family can be pushed from "just getting by" into the lack of adequate care that constitutes neglect.

Dubowitz (1999) urges us to focus on the child's unmet needs rather than on parental wrongdoing when we try to determine if a child has been neglected. David Hamburg (1992), president of the Carnegie Corporation Foundation, condemned U.S. society for its "collective neglect" in failing to provide policies that support families in caring for children, and in failing to provide adequate healthcare, childcare, preschool education, and housing for families. In the United States and Canada, there is a confounding of social class with ethnic and racial factors, so that higher percentages of African Americans, Native Americans, and Latinos fall below the poverty line as compared to Whites. In addition, even within a large ethnic category that looks fairly stable economically, such as Asian Americans, there are pockets of great poverty, such as among Cambodians and recent Chinese immigrants, who may live and work in extremely unfavorable conditions. Poor children are more likely to be removed from their home for issues of maltreatment than middle-class or wealthy children and, once removed, African American children are less likely than children of other races to be reunited with their families or adopted (Charlow, 2001–2002). That is, once they are removed from their homes African American children are more likely to stay in foster care or institutions until adulthood. Charlow (2001–2002) urges us to apply the imminent-danger-of-harm standard before making placement decisions. Where possible, we should offer support to keep families intact and safe, not placement.

How do we, as child maltreatment professionals, handle the poverty-related issues that we face daily in our work? In some cases our hands are tied and we may feel forced to work at the individual level even though we recognize that change needs to happen at a wider social level. We may have the ability and training to remove a child from his home but not to assure his family a more adequate income. However, sometimes the resources of the child's proximal social systems can add enough support to the family to help them provide adequately for their child, and avoid the disruption caused by out-of-home placement.

Armstrong (1995) writes that we co-opt, defuse, and manage the social/political problems we encounter "by reformulating them as mental health problems . . . this language tends to paralyze our critical skills and deflect attention from compelling social problems" (p. 25). When we find out a child has been hurt, we open a case file and seek an individual or family solution: foster care, parenting classes, psychotherapy, or often simply continued monitoring by state agencies. The links between inadequate resources for families and child maltreatment seem clear and paramount to me, and yet it is easier to seek and implement individual solutions, hoping to save a tree as we watch the forest burn.

When I was working as a psychotherapist in a community agency, my clients were often poor single mothers who lacked adequate housing, employment, childcare, and healthcare. I could easily understand how, in this context, they had hurt or neglected their children—the pressures of their life circumstances easily overwhelmed their ability to cope. And yet often the best I could offer them was psychotherapy. Eliminating poverty would undoubtedly go a long way in reducing child abuse and neglect by reducing family stress, providing wider support networks, and increasing resources for all families. I hope people who work to eliminate maltreatment will also pursue the broader goal of eliminating poverty.

## CHILD MALTREATMENT

The term "child maltreatment" encompasses both *child abuse* (willful acts that harm a child including sexual, physical, and emotional abuse) and *neglect* (failure to provide for a child's basic needs). Clearly, this definition leaves much room for interpretation. How to distinguish between milder forms of maltreatment and suboptimal parenting is beyond the scope of this chapter, and may indeed be impossible. There are many situations where children's spirits are crushed by harsh words and their bodies worn out by harsh actions, but these do not meet the standards for intervention by child protection authorities. We who work with families must find ways to support families and children in situations of maltreatment *and* in situations of suboptimal parenting to help foster the best possible conditions for children. That is, beyond the question of whether they "need to be reported" to child protection authorities, or whether children need to be placed in safer homes, many families will benefit from caring support and information. When we think of ourselves as resources to help all families, then the question of when to report becomes a side issue (one reports when one has suspicion of child abuse and neglect, period). Our responsibility to help families neither begins nor ends with the report (see Chapter 3).

The labeling of a given act as "maltreatment" necessarily involves cultural components and value judgments (see Chapters 3 and 5). I decline the temptation to develop a single, universal definition of child maltreatment. Rather, I am using this book to explore multiple takes on the concept of child maltreatment, and to address how we can improve the fairness of the child welfare system.

## WORKING WITH FAMILIES

In accord with the ecosystemic framework I discussed above, agencies should assess their ability to serve families as a whole, and not just individuals. Here I'll make a brief plea for the importance of involving the children's families in our approach. While limited contacts with professionals such as psychotherapists and social workers constitute part of a child's recovery environment, a far larger part of this environment is made up of the child's family. Only through consistent work with the child victim's family can professionals make sure that a child will have the best possible recovery environment and avoid future episodes of abuse. (By "family," here, I am referring either to the child's original family, or the child's new family, in a situation where parental rights have been terminated.)

Professionals have a great ability to influence the long-term response of family members to a child's maltreatment: whether the child will be ostracized or supported, believed or disbelieved, cast as a villain or as a brave hero for speaking up, and protected or subjected to further abuse. Family interventions are apt to be key to a child's long-term recovery (indeed, a primary predictor of a girl's recovery from incest is whether her mother believes the disclosure [Elliott & Carnes, 2001]). For these reasons, we must find ways to engage families in our work. Many mental health professionals have been trained in individual approaches, and they may be more comfortable conducting play therapy with a single victim, for instance, than engaging in sessions with an unruly and unpredictable family. But we need to remember that the family rather than the individual is the central unit in many cultures, and therefore family work resonates especially well with families from most cultural groups.

A thorough discussion of family approaches to child abuse is certainly beyond the scope of this book; however, excellent resources are available (see Gil, 1996a; Trepper & Barrett, 1989). Below I briefly discuss some strategies that may be helpful in working with families from diverse groups and for making our work user-friendly to all families.

## Who's Who?: Acquiring Demographic Information

Sometimes we meet families after reading a thick case folder about them. At other times we have little advance material. Often the background information we have been given is at least partially incorrect. Gathering basic demographic information can be complicated, especially when the interviewer and the family come from different cultural backgrounds.

Many families do not fit the nuclear model of mom, dad, and the kids. For example, extended family members and grown siblings may live at home with the child or in an apartment down the hall. Close family friends may be called "aunts" and "uncles" and live with the family for a time, although they are not related by blood or marriage (these are called "fictive kin"). Aunts, uncles, godparents, and grandparents may serve as children's caretakers and wield as much influence over the children as their own parents. Children may float between various households within their extended families, going to grandma's after school, eating dinner at their aunt's, and sometimes sleeping at their godparents' home. Social workers can be confused by such arrangements if they are checking the food supply in Mom's refrigerator and find that it is empty—but her children actually take their meals in another household.

Boyd-Franklin (2003) describes many variations of informal adoptions that occur in some African American families, as extended family members and family friends may help each other out in a tight spot by welcoming another person's child to live in their household. Some of the circumstances she describes include when older relatives raise the child of a teen mother so she can pursue her education; when relatives or friends in a good school district allow a youngster to live with them to permit him or her to attend a better school; and when a mother is going through a hard time economically or has lost her housing and other relatives care for the child until the mother has established a new home. Sometimes mothers are forced to give up their children to pursue their education or to attend drug or alcohol treatment. While this flexibility of households often works successfully as an unofficial support system for families who may be living on the economic edge, occasionally changes in circumstances and expectations may result in custody battles and other complications.

We need to ask questions in ways that allow the respondents to acknowledge gay and lesbian partners, children conceived outside of marriage, informal adoptions, and common-law spouses. We should remember that the words "Daddy" or "Papi" might be used to describe a biological father, a stepfather, a grandfather, the mother's boyfriend, or another important male in the child's life. The child may say he lives with Mama but he knows Mama is his grandmother and he visits Mommy on weekends. In families from India, Pakistan, and Bangladesh, any older female friend of the family is apt to be called "Auntie." Because of China's one-child policy, some Chinese youngsters describe children their own age as "brothers" and "sisters" when in fact they are cousins or neighbors. In Chinese and Native American families, people may be called "cousins" because they come from the same tribe or ancestral village.

The possibilities of relationships and living arrangements are endless. We must be open to hearing about each child's reality, not as we imagine it but as the child actually lives it. Similarly, paperwork should have categories that are inclusive to gay men and lesbians, informal adoptive families, extended families that live together, and so on (see Chapter 2 for a discussion of translating paperwork).

Among Latin cultures including the Latin American, Spanish, Portuguese, and Italian ones, godparents are often considered family, although there is usually no blood relationship. When a parent names a person his child's godfather or godmother, he enters into a codified relationship with that person, and they are called in Spanish *compadres* or *comadres* (literally, co-fathers or co-mothers). In these cultures, if a godparent sexually abuses a godchild, it may have the impact of incest.

In addition, in many cultures a marriage does not merely join two individuals, but rather it joins two extended families (illustrated vividly and humorously in the movie *My Big Fat Greek Wedding*). In some cultures, the relationships between the in-laws are dignified with a name—in Spanish, the in-laws become *consuegros* (literally "co-in-laws") and in Yiddish the two extended families become *mishpucha*. The fact that English does not have special names for these relationships shows their relative lack of importance in cultures that use the English language. When we work with diverse families we should make sure our vision of who the family is (and, possibly, therefore, who should be included in assessment and treatment) encompasses *all* relevant people.

## Joining with All Members of the Family

Some families will want to include extended family members and godparents in all interactions with professionals. Sometimes you might want to challenge interaction patterns that appear to be dysfunctional, and some of these may involve members of the extended family. However, if you approach a family in a challenging way too soon, there may be no chance to establish a solid working relationship later on (Trepper & Barrett, 1989). Sometimes, when a particular individual has been identified as the "problem" (e.g., an incestuous father), one of his relatives (e.g., his mother) may have been told to watch over the family in their interactions with professionals. I encourage you to welcome members of the family into your work who have been chosen by the child's caretakers, but you may still need to have separate conversations with family members to assess for risk and understand the family's dynamics.

In most families, it will be helpful to honor the hierarchy by first greeting the older members of the family (parents or perhaps even grandparents), and then asking them to introduce the children. Often, it will be helpful to acknowledge the father first. (However, in some cultural groups, such as among the Amish, female professionals will be considered disrespectful if they address adult male family members directly. Men will typically attend important family meetings with their wives and children, but if the professional is female, they may "watch over" the session, rather than participate.) In this topic, as in so many others, true familiarity with the culture will enable us to figure out the appropriate way to proceed.

## Addressing Clients Properly

We need to find out how the child and family members like to be addressed. Many Spanish, Portuguese, Italian, and southern United States names are double names, such as María Teresa, José Antonio, or Mary Sue. My eldest daughter's name is Ana Lua, and she always introduces herself this way. Whenever an adult replies with "Hi, Ana," she feels cut off from this person—who didn't really bother to listen to her name or try to get it right. Of course many children are called by their nicknames. Make sure you address children in their preferred way, saying the name a few times if necessary until you can pronounce it correctly.

Chinese names usually begin with the surname and end with what is called the first name in the West. So someone whose name is written "Lo En Chen" should be addressed as "Mrs. Lo"—not necessarily what you'd expect.

In Russian and other Slavic cultures, names may have different endings depending on whether the person is male or female. That is, almost every female first name ends in "a," female middle names end in "ovna," and female last names end in "ova," "ovna," or "skaya." Middle names are actually patronymics, meaning that they are formed from the father's first name with "ovna" appended. For example, a girl whose American name is Lucy, but is the daughter of Alexander Popov, would be Lucya Alexandrovna Popova. Libby, the daughter of Vladimir Putin, would be Luba Vladimirovna Putina. One thing that may be confusing about this for people less familiar with Slavic cultures is that all the boys in a family will share a middle and last name, as do all the girls. And the girls and the boys in the same family will have different last names, since the girls have the endings appended. Some Russian and Slavic families have adopted the naming traditions of their new countries and have dropped the gendered endings on their names. It can be hard for people who are less familiar with the culture to keep all this straight. But it's important to be aware of these possibilities, and to try our best.

When speaking with adults, it is important to address them by their last names, as Mr. or Ms. whomever, rather than assuming the familiarity of using first names. Particularly when working with older people who are from an oppressed group, such as African Americans, the familiarity of the first name might seem like an insult. For generations White people addressed African Americans by their first names, while expecting to be addressed as "Sir" or "Ma'am" in return. Therefore, older African Americans may feel insulted when professionals use first names with them.

As egalitarian as we may try to be, the professional is the one who holds the power in the encounter. This reminds me of when I saw my new dentist for the first time. He is a relatively young man who—without asking my permission—started calling me by my first name. He shook my hand and said, "Hi, Lisa, I'm Dr. Carver." This imbalance in forms of address felt demeaning and I was already intimidated enough just by being there! He held the potential to inflict pain on me, so I did not argue with his presentation. Clients in the child maltreatment system feel the same way. We can ask to be addressed by our first names, if we so choose, but we should not assume this familiarity with adult clients unless they indicate that they too would like to be addressed by their first names.

## Conveying Respect

We must do our best to convey respect to family members. Becoming involved in the child protection system and all its many components is often embarrassing and even humiliating for families. We need to do what we can to help families maintain and recover their dignity. How do we know if we are behaving in a way that is respectful? We pay careful attention to what we say and how we present ourselves, and then do a "topsy-turvy" and try to figure out *how our clients hear us*. "Topsy-turvies are illustrations that when turned 180 degrees display two completely different images. For example, a topsy-turvy might look like a smiling woman from one perspective but when turned 180 degrees it might look like a nasty and angry pirate" (Kohl, 2002, p. 150). To be able to try on our clients' shoes, we need to accept the idea of a mismatch between the way we *want* to be seen and heard and the image that we are actually conveying. We must examine how we pose questions, explain regulations, look inside bedrooms, search apartments, examine injuries, fill out forms—and we should explore how these activities may feel from the client's end. As we catch ourselves conveying any trace of disrespect, we must have the courage to try something new. In our professional roles we may still need to do things our clients would rather we did not do, but a respectful attitude can make these actions easier to accept.

## Accessing Resources for Families

Professionals must serve as a social intermediary or matchmaker between families and community institutions (Falicov, 1996, p. 174), particularly when those families are from immigrant or ethnic minority groups and may not trust or be familiar with available services. Social isolation is one of the greatest risk factors for child maltreatment.

Effective intervention requires a coordinated response. We need to reach out to child protection professionals, community and religious leaders, spiritual healers, physicians, nurses, teachers, law enforcement officers, attorneys, counselors, people who work in women's shelters, and others. Even with our limited budgets it is a necessity, not a luxury, to meet with these people for lunch or coffee or an exchange of ideas. We should get to know them before we need to ask them for a favor. These people can serve as sources of referrals, and may be able to help in our work with specific families.

# RESEARCH AND CLINICAL LITERATURE
# ON CULTURE AND CHILD MALTREATMENT

The literature on cultural minority groups and child maltreatment is contradictory and inadequate. The rates of child abuse reported in community samples is remarkably similar across ethnic groups (Charlow, 2001–2002). However, we know that African American, Native American, and Latin American children are overrepresented in the child welfare system generally, in *reported* cases of child maltreatment, and in foster care, as compared to their percentages in the population at large, and even their representation among people of lower income (Chipungu & Bent-Goodley, 2003; Roberts, 2002; U.S. Department of Health and Human Services, Administration for Children and Families, 2002). In recent national reporting statistics (U.S. Department of Health and Human Services, Administration for Children and Families, 2002) African American children comprised 26% of reported cases (they are 12% of the child population), Hispanic children 11% (they are 13% of the child population), Native Americans and Alaskan Native children 2% (they are 0.7% of the child population), and Asian Pacific Islander children 1% (they are 4% of the child population).[3] On the other hand, Whites and Asian Americans are found to be *underrepresented* in the child welfare and foster care systems, as compared to their proportion of the general population. The causes of these differences in representation are hotly debated. Possibilities include true differences in maltreatment levels based on differences in poverty levels, cultural differences, or neighborhood deterioration (Coulton, Korbin, & Su, 1999); biases in the reporting, substantiating, and handling of suspected child abuse (Ards, Chung, & Myers, 1998); and lack of social services and outreach in certain communities. Once racial and ethnic minority parents fall into the child welfare system, the interventions are more likely to be adversarial, as indicated by a greater number of civil and criminal court proceedings (Tjaden & Thoennes, 1992; Roberts, 2002).

Until this recent surge of interest in culture (and still today, for the most part), research on child abuse has simply ignored issues of cultural variability, assuming that all families are the same (e.g., like White families). Researchers often "controlled for ethnicity" by using all-White samples (e.g., Herman, 1981), failing to report the ethnicity of the people studied (e.g., Ligezinska et al., 1996), or reporting the ethnic mix of the sample but failing to assess for group differences in reporting the results (e.g., Barnett, Martinez, & Keyson, 1996). Comparative studies are often marred by dividing groups into categories that are poorly conceived,

---

[3]Although Asian American children are underrepresented in national statistics, this finding does not always hold in geographical areas with high concentrations of Asian Americans, and reporting rates vary by country of origin.

in what I have termed "ethnic lumping" (Fontes, 1995a). That is, researchers might classify Japanese and Pakistani Americans as "Asian Americans," failing to assess for differences between these two groups. Or researchers might lump together people who have the same national or ethnic origin but who have been in this country for differing generations, and are therefore likely to have widely varied concerns, such as sixth-generation Chinese Americans and Chinese who arrived from Hong Kong last month.

In another form of ethnic lumping, researchers overgeneralize when they use a category such as "Latino" to describe the part of their sample that consists wholly of Mexican Americans. It is incorrect to assume that the results would apply to all Latinos. Sometimes researchers fail to distinguish between race and social class (Lockhart, 1985) or culture and poverty (Zayas, 1992).

Most of the clinical literature in the field is written by members of the dominant group, and—like the research literature—similarly ignores issues of culture. The number of students and faculty of color in professional schools continues to be low, and training in multicultural issues tends to be spotty at best. Although typically one finds greater cultural diversity the lower one descends in the professional status hierarchy, supervisors and researchers are more likely to be White and middle or upper middle class. This affects the expectations and stereotypes they bring to their writing and thinking about cultural issues in child abuse, and therefore has an impact on the field.

Starting in the mid-1990s, research and treatment literature began to emerge focusing on cultural issues in child maltreatment in North America. These works range from full-length books on cultural issues in abuse (Fontes, 1995a; Lewis, 1999; Stone, 2004; Wilson, 1994) to research articles that analyze results for ethnicity (Beahl, Crouch, May, Valente, & Conyngham, 2001) to analyses of particular issues in particular groups (e.g., Mosby, Rawls, Meehan, Mays, & Pettinari, 1999), many of which are cited throughout this book.

The recent interest in cultural issues in child maltreatment may be attributed to the maturation of the field. While there still is much to learn, our notions of maltreatment have become more textured and precise. We are able to make distinctions between the long- and short-term effects of different types of abuse, for instance, and tailor our treatment plans accordingly. We have treatment protocols that differ according to the family structure and the victim's age, developmental level, and gender. Similarly, we are recognizing the need to work with families in ways that respect and honor their whole selves, including their cultures.

Gender roles, religious beliefs, views of virginity, disciplinary practices, and a host of other cultural norms together shape a person's experience of maltreatment. Additionally, culture will determine the kind of help—if any—that a victim will accept to cope with the abuse. Culture is a building block of self-identity. As such a fundamental part of who we are, culture cannot be ignored in designing interventions for child abuse and neglect.

## CONCLUDING THOUGHTS: REMEMBERING THE DIFFICULTY OF THE MATERIAL AND THE SACREDNESS OF OUR WORK

Many of us work with issues of child abuse every day. Over time, without even realizing it, we may become numb to histories of suffering and cruelty. In its extreme form, this is a kind of "burnout" and interferes with our work. In a mild form, it's just a way to cope. We may tell morbid jokes. We may breathe a sigh of relief when we find out that a child we are working with has "only" been abused physically and not sexually, or that a child is a victim of "garden-variety sexual abuse" with "only" one perpetrator. We may forget that the teenager who was raped "just once" was still violated and is in crisis. We may overlook the fear on the face of a child who has been beaten because this situation seems so much simpler, more straightforward, and milder than the sadistic case we handled yesterday. We may downplay the importance of some indicators of neglect and prefer not to investigate any further because we just cannot take on another case or bear to hear another tale of suffering.

Speaking about child maltreatment in any way is taboo in some cultures. When we inquire about a family's practices and a child's well-being, when we ask questions about sleeping arrangements, eating, hygiene, sexual practices, and discipline, we are within inches of a terrain that the family may consider too intimate to discuss. Saba and Rodgers (1990) tell the tragic story of a Cambodian man who brought his son into the emergency room with a fever of 103 degrees. The father seemed anxious and spoke little English. Upon exam, the physician saw bruising across the child's back, assumed it was due to abuse, and called child protective services to report possible child abuse. The doctor admitted the child to the hospital and sent the father home. The father hung himself that night, ashamed that he had "lost" his son and that the authorities thought badly of him. It turned out the bruises resulted from coining (see Chapter 2) and not abuse. Clearly, a Cambodian interpreter would have been essential here. But in addition, the physician seemed to have lost touch with the enormous force of his actions and the father's vulnerability. We must never forget the power of our words and actions.

Steele (1989) has called psychotherapy with survivors of sexual abuse "sitting with the shattered soul," and I think the same concept can be applied to all work with people involved in family violence. The police officer who arrests a drunk and violent parent, the physician who attends to a bruised child, the social worker who inquires about prior incidents, the psychologist who asks a child if she feels safe, the attorney or forensic interviewer who is assessing a child's statement—each of these professionals is working with a person who has undergone a difficult or traumatic experience, and each of these professionals is entering into a noble relationship with the client. It may not feel that way, but we need to remember the sacredness of this encounter and the difficulty of the material for the client.

Why do I use words like "noble" and "sacred" in a book on cultural competency? "Sacred" pertains to the idea of reverence or respect, attitudes we must bring to our every professional interaction, and particularly with those who are from a social group that is stigmatized in our country. If we convey an understanding of the seriousness of our endeavor, and the pain involved, our clients from diverse backgrounds are more likely to trust us. We are more likely to build the kind of working relationship that will allow us to do our best work: keeping children safe while respecting families and their cultures.

## QUESTIONS TO THINK ABOUT AND DISCUSS

1. What is the ecosystemic framework and how does it apply to issues of child maltreatment?

2. Describe some of the ways your professional culture and your ethnic culture are the same, and some ways they are different.

3. How might prejudice and stereotyping affect professional decision making in child maltreatment? Describe a time when you saw this occur.

4. Describe how poverty relates to child maltreatment.

5. What are some of the reasons that a family from an oppressed cultural group might reject your sincere attempts to help?

# CHAPTER TWO

# Working with Immigrant Families Affected by Child Maltreatment

This chapter provides information on how the experience of immigration itself can affect family life and particularly child welfare. It also describes ways to intervene effectively in child abuse and neglect across cultural and linguistic differences. In the year 2003, 20% of children in the United States were found to have at least one foreign-born parent (Federal Interagency Forum on Child and Family Statistics, 2004).

## SOCIAL STRESSORS FOR IMMIGRANT FAMILIES

Immigrants to the United States and Canada are widely diverse, ranging from highly educated professionals who speak English fluently, hold white-collar jobs, and are well integrated into the dominant culture, to people who are illiterate, undocumented, unemployed, speak no English, and may be marginalized in every way. Of course, most people who immigrate to North America fall somewhere in between these two extremes.

The process of immigration can place people in puzzling situations. Political changes may force a rural peasant from Somalia or Guatemala to flee his homeland overnight, thrusting him suddenly into a large North American city where his centuries-old skills in village social relations and farming are useless and unmarketable. Or a prominent dentist from the big city of Bogotá, Colombia, may come to North America in search of a safer environment for her children, finding after arriving that her dental license is not valid here, and that she has to work as a janitor, with coworkers who treat her as a "dumb foreigner."

Even when migration has been carefully planned, its effects can be gravely disorienting. My in-laws immigrated to the United States from Portugal when they were in their mid-50s. My husband was able to find them steady work almost immediately. Although my father-in-law's age and poor hearing interfered with his ability to learn English, by all criteria he seemed to be adjusting well to his new homeland. Nevertheless, 10 years after he'd immigrated my mother-in-law confessed to me that my father-in-law was still so uncomfortable handling U.S. money, and felt so diminished by his lack of English skills at the checkout counter, that he refused to buy even a quart of milk without his wife. Clearly, the psychological effects of immigrating had made him powerless in ways we did not imagine and had radically altered both his self-image and his personal relationships.

The disruptive effects of immigration cannot be overestimated. The greater the difference between the culture of origin and the new environment, the longer lasting the resulting culture shock is apt to be. This chapter primarily concerns those immigrants who are less well acculturated, and who therefore may present the greatest challenge to professionals unfamiliar with the beliefs and behaviors they have brought with them from their countries of origin.

## Culture Shock and Disruption

*Culture shock* may be defined as the anxiety and disorientation people feel as they try to adjust to a culture that is different from the one they are used to. Since culture shock distorts almost every aspect of daily life for recent immigrants, it may complicate efforts to obtain an accurate assessment of parenting. Immigrant families face cultural differences from the moment they wake up to a foreign voice on the radio to the moment they go to sleep in an unfamiliar room. The need to learn a new language can be overwhelming, particularly for older adults and for those who have had little formal schooling. Some people simply refuse to learn the language of their new country, believing that to do so would in some way betray their ties to their country of origin. For others, their effort to express themselves in a new language is a constant source of stress and feelings of inadequacy.

Daily interactions with people outside the ethnic group can be a continual source of anxiety. Immigrants may try to smooth out relationships by smiling and nodding convincingly, even though they understand little of what is being said. Immigrants are often confused by their interactions with institutions such as schools, courts, hospitals, banks, and housing and immigration authorities, which may differ dramatically from those agencies "back home." Immigrant families who are undocumented live in constant fear of deportation. And political refugees must cope with the after-effects of the trauma they have suffered.

Moving to the United States or Canada can cause families' traditional gender roles to unravel, provoking temporary periods of stress and conflict until family members settle into new roles. Women who may never have had paid employment sometimes become the sole breadwinners in the new country, leaving them exhausted and their family members resentful. Immigrant men who are unable to find paid employment, or who are forced to work at jobs where they are demeaned and exploited, may become angry or depressed, and turn to gambling, alcohol, drugs, or violence to help them cope.

Or the opposite may happen. Women who have been lively and active members of their communities, engaging in paid work outside the home or contributing to the family's livelihood through farming or selling wares at the market, may become isolated and homebound in their new countries. This has occurred among many of the Somali refugee families who have recently moved into my area. The women typically stay home and do not attend English lessons. Ostensibly this is because the women have young children and must stay at home to care for them. In Somalia, however, women continue to engage in public life throughout their pregnancies and the rearing of young children; they bring their children with them. I am fearful about the future of this generation of refugee women who are not learning to speak English and who are remaining vastly less acculturated than their husbands and children. I do not know how they will fend for themselves if they become widowed or are separated from their husbands. Even if their families stay intact, their contributions to the family income are apt to be needed once their public benefits have expired, and they lack even the most minimal language skills. I also worry about their psychological well-being if they remain unable to communicate in their new land.

A certain degree of paranoia is not uncommon among immigrant families. It may endure for years in the absence of intervention from caring neighbors or professionals. The immigrants have lost their "road maps," they do not know what is expected of them in daily interactions, and they are frightened about the dangers that may lurk in unknown places. An immigrant man who is experiencing paranoia may restrain his wife and children in ways that seem incomprehensible—perhaps refusing to allow them to leave the home, answer the phone, or attend after-school activities. When professionals encounter this kind of behavior, they need to ask questions about the family's functioning prior to immigration to ascertain whether these current behaviors were practiced in the country of origin or if they have been adopted in response to the stresses of migration. In either case, a family needs to be helped to function in ways that allow each of its members a measure of self-determination and freedom from exploitation and control, while still respecting the family's deeply held values.

## Isolation

In one of her brilliant short stories about the life of South Asian immigrants in the United States, Jhumpa Lahiri (1999, p. 116) presents a conversation between a recent Indian immigrant who is the wife of a college professor and the 11-year-old boy whom she cares for after school each day:

> "Eliot, if I began to scream right now at the top of my lungs, would someone come?"
>
> "Mrs. Sen, what's wrong?"
>
> "Nothing. I am only asking if someone would come."
>
> Eliot shrugged. "Maybe."
>
> "At home, that is all you have to do. Not everybody has a telephone. But just raise your voice a bit, or express grief or joy of any kind, and one whole neighborhood and half of another has come to share the news, to help with arrangements."
>
> By then Eliot understood that when Mrs. Sen said home, she meant India, not the apartment where she sat chopping vegetables.

Migration has an isolating effect on many immigrant families. Some immigrant families move back and forth to their countries of origin every few years. Others, especially refugees, may have made a single traumatic break with their native land. They may have lost forever the possibility of returning home or of maintaining contact with friends, family, and even spouses and children in their native countries. Many immigrants move repeatedly within the United States or Canada in search of better employment, education, housing, healthcare, or social service benefits. When children are uprooted a number of times, they are less likely to develop strong ties with people they can trust in their communities.

Many immigrant children sense early on the vulnerability of their most trusted relatives. "How can Mami protect me from our neighbor," the child of an immigrant might wonder, "if she needs me to read her mail and answer the phone?" Although I have not seen research on this topic, I have noticed that sexual molesters sometimes deliberately prey upon immigrant children because they perceive the children's isolation and consequent vulnerability.

One therapist told me that when he works with a child who has been sexually molested, he tries to identify a family member whom the child can trust, and then uses this person as an ally in therapy. However, he has found this practice more difficult to accomplish with immigrant families because the most trusted family members may not be in this country, but rather may remain in the country of origin (Fontes, 1993b).

Discrimination also isolates immigrant families. Unless they are personally close to immigrants, native-born Americans may find it hard to understand the far reach and dire effects of anti-immigrant sentiment. I knew an immigrant who worked as a janitor at a university. When he was transferred from an office building to a dormitory, he was regularly harassed by a group of football players on one floor who seemed to enjoy taunting him. They would upturn garbage cans in front of him and smear feces in the bathrooms. He endured such treatment for months before his son helped him complain to his supervisor. He did not understand that official avenues of redress were available to him. Besides, he mistrusted the university authorities. For 2 months he had cleaned a chemistry laboratory before he was informed that he was working in the presence of radioactive materials that required special precautions. His employers could not find an interpreter to teach him the necessary safety training, so they did not bother to alert him to the radioactive dangers, nor did they tell him how to protect himself. When he found out about the missed safety training and his supervisors' lack of concern for his well-being, he lost his faith in them as sources of help or support.

Immigrants are often subjected to discrimination by the very organizations that are charged with protecting and caring for them, such as school, police, legal, and social service personnel. Although teachers and school counselors can be key players in the prevention and detection of child abuse, children will refuse to confide in them if they perceive the school as an alien or even a hostile place. Many immigrant children have been taught to fear people who represent "the system." One Puerto Rican woman told me proudly that she had instructed her children *never* to go to the school nurse. The mother believed that the nurse was prejudiced against Latinos, and so she told her children, "I don't care how sick you are. If you talk to that lady I'm not going to come pick you up." In her attempt to protect her children and herself from prejudice, this mother was actually isolating her children.

When professionals carry a bias against people who do not speak English well, or who request an interpreter, they serve to further isolate their immigrant clients. At a talk I gave recently, one social worker stated that some colleagues at her agency believe that their immigrant clients actually speak English better than they are letting on, and that they are pretending they don't speak English to get some sort of special treatment. "Why," she asked, "would anyone possibly pretend he doesn't speak a language if he were capable of expressing himself in that language?" Like this social worker, I cannot imagine any secondary gain to be derived from feigning a limited ability to speak English. Rather, I think her colleagues were mistaking the clients' ability to "get by" in English for greater English-speaking skills than they actually possess. We should work hard to provide whatever bilingual or interpreting services might be necessary so people with limited English proficiency can feel as comfortable using our services as other people.

After the social worker spoke, a police officer chimed in, "I can do you one better! In my department the chief won't assign Spanish-speaking officers to Spanish-speaking neighborhoods, because he thinks it will be good for the Latin American immigrants to be forced to speak English. He doesn't seem to understand that when they can't communicate with the police easily, people just run away from us."

I empathize with the officer's frustration. An encounter with a police officer is not an opportunity to practice language skills. Anything less than providing the best possible police protection to *all* residents is discriminatory, possibly illegal, and certainly not compassionate.

Lack of telephones and transportation also isolates many low-income immigrant children from potential sources of support. Children who live in neighborhoods marred by crime and violence may not be allowed to visit friends and relatives, even if they live within walking distance. Lack of health insurance may also lead poor families to rely on emergency rooms rather than a family physician, thus cutting them off from another adult who might notice a change in their behaviors, or whom they might otherwise trust with a disclosure.

We should work to reduce the isolation of immigrant families. Extended family members, godparents, neighbors, friends, teachers, and clergy may be able to provide physical and emotional support to families, and may even serve as formal or informal foster parents when necessary. Sometimes a teacher or a school counselor can be enlisted to watch over or to meet regularly with a child. Reducing parental isolation through parent aides, English tutors, vocational or reading classes, and contacts with religious or civic organizations is also likely to benefit children.

## FAMILY LIFE, CHILD BEHAVIOR, AND DISCIPLINE

For many immigrants, family is a source of pride, strength, identity, and help, as it was in their country of origin. But during the process of immigration, families may literally be torn apart. Family members may not immigrate all at the same time. The children may be left behind in the country of origin until the parents are settled, or the children may be sent to the new country first to live with an extended family member while the parents work to obtain the necessary money or visas to join them. While these atypical family configurations are often safe and loving, occasionally this distance from their parents exposes children to greater risk of physical or sexual abuse.

In Latino families, it is not uncommon for a father to migrate first, while the mother stays in Mexico or Puerto Rico with her children, supported by members of her extended family (Falicov, 1998). The family reorganizes around the father's absence, and subsequently may undergo considerable distress when they eventually move to the new country and try to adapt to the father's presence again. Some fathers become rigid and even violent in attempting to reassert their position in the family.

Triandis (1994) has proposed that cultures are divided into those that are *individualist*, emphasizing autonomy, individuality, and independence, and those that are *collectivist*, emphasizing family loyalty, closeness, interdependence, affiliation, and cooperation. The dominant cultures in the United States and Canada are considered individualist, whereas the dominant cultures in much of Latin America, Africa, southern Europe, and Asia are considered collectivist. When the child of an immigrant learns individualist values in school and through the mass media, and brings them home to a collectivist household, intergenerational tension commonly results. In extreme cases, this conflict can result in child abuse. For example, a teenager who insists that it is more important to do his homework or attend a friend's party than to accompany a family member to the airport may be viewed as selfish and uncaring, and punished accordingly.

Above all, immigrant parents want their children to be safe and protected. This may be particularly true of recent immigrants who are bewildered by all the potential dangers of their new country. They are unlikely to leave their young children with caretakers other than family members, even when professionals might believe the child would be better off in an established childcare center than at home with a member of the extended family. If you believe current childcare arrangements are unsound in a given family, it may be important to explain carefully and in great detail the advantages of a childcare center for this particular child at this particular time (e.g., increased opportunities to prepare for school, access to stimulating activities rather than television, social interactions in the English language). Alternatively, you may want to facilitate the training and credentialing of the informal caregiver as a licensed childcare provider.

Immigrants often feel that their welcome in their new country is contingent on their being as invisible and compliant as possible. For this reason, many immigrants insist that their children behave impeccably in public. Unlike many White native-born parents who prefer to keep up a conflict-free public image, immigrant parents who observe their children acting disobediently or disrespectfully in public may respond immediately with a cutting comment or a blow, placing them at greater risk for reports to child protection authorities.

Many traditional immigrant families may use an authoritarian style of parenting, demanding total obedience and respect from their children. While these practices do not necessarily constitute child abuse, they are apt to clash with the child-rearing norms of mainstream U.S. and Canadian culture, and may bring the parents to the attention of the child protection system. Additionally, studies consistently establish a link between both familial and neighborhood poverty and neglect or physical child abuse, also increasing the likelihood that child abuse professionals will have low-income immigrants in their caseload.

Many immigrant parents expect their children to follow orders. Caribbean parents, for instance, tend to be more strict and authoritarian than both U.S. White and Black parents (Payne, 1989). When children of Caribbean parents disobey, their parents often respond harshly, sometimes resorting to corporal punishment. Educated Caribbean parents are likely to speak with their children *and* to use corporal punishment. Less-educated parents may simply respond punitively. The more educated and acculturated the family is, the closer its child discipline norms may be to those of the mainstream culture. Whether an immigrant family's corporal punishment constitutes physical abuse depends on its frequency and severity and the impact it has on the child (see Chapter 5).

## IMMIGRANTS AND THE CHILD WELFARE SYSTEM

The child protection system in the United States is, for the most part, cruelly unfair to immigrant parents. This is not a criticism of the individuals who work in the system but rather of the system as a whole. Fortunately, many dedicated professionals are working to improve it.

Immigrant parents often do not know what is expected of them, but they are still punished when they fail to comply with unwritten cultural expectations. Language and cultural barriers have always made it difficult for immigrant families to access services. But today the isolation of immigrant families is compounded by recent federal and state laws that restrict immigrants' eligibility for certain services. The 1996 federal welfare and immigration laws in the United States, coupled with harsh anti-immigrant sentiment and legislation enacted in response to the September 11, 2001, World Trade Center and Pentagon attacks, have made many immigrants worry about endangering themselves by contacting government agencies. Those laws have also made many immigrant families fear that if they or their children use any government services, this might negatively impact their immigration status. They often fear that the benefits agency will share information about their family with immigration authorities. This fear applies not only to undocumented immigrants and people seeking refugee status, but also to legal immigrants who want to renew their permanent resident status (green card), to change from permanent resident to citizen status, or to sponsor relatives to come to the United States.

There seems to be a backlash today against giving needed help to immigrant families. The U.S. myth of self-sufficiency and "pulling yourself up by your own bootstraps" is being applied wholesale to immigrants and refugees. State and local governments are making drastic cuts in bilingual education, social services, and healthcare for documented and undocumented aliens and for citizens who are children of the foreign-born, without compassion for the immigrant families and without facing up to the impact of these cuts on the nation as a whole.

The vision of the United States as a welcoming refuge for one and all—as symbolized by the Statue of Liberty—seems to have been cast aside. Citizens whose families have been in this country for several generations seem to forget that the government supported *their* ancestors when they settled here decades ago. No immigrant group that has settled successfully in North America ever accomplished this entirely "on their own," without help from those who came before them. Immigrant children and families need supports and specialized services until they gain the skills to survive and thrive in the dominant culture.

## Neglect Issues for Immigrants

Low-income immigrant parents are vulnerable to charges of neglect that stem from lack of acculturation to U.S. and Canadian norms. For instance, parents may be penalized for leaving their children home alone or allowing them to play unsupervised in the street, even though this was the norm in their communities of origin, where neighbors watched out for each others' children. Rogoff (2003) documents that supervision by siblings is the norm in many cultures, and can be highly beneficial for children's development. In many cultural settings, although siblings and older children may be doing the direct supervising, adults will be within earshot. In the U.S. or Canadian context, however, children who are left for even short periods of time without an adult's supervision may be seen as "neglected" depending on their age and circumstances. Faced with this backdrop, before undertaking any other intervention, professionals need to assess and affirm immigrant parents' substantial efforts to educate and provide for their children despite difficult circumstances. Educating parents about the norms of the new country is apt to be more helpful than a punishing response.

Automobiles represent another source of potential conflict for which well-meaning immigrant parents might be found neglectful. Many immigrants to the United States and Canada come from poor communities and are not familiar with the responsibilities inherent in owning a car in their new country. For instance, they may believe it is cruel to allow a child to cry alone in a rear car seat, believing it is more caring to cradle the child in their arms. They may not understand the cultural proscription against leaving a child alone in a car for brief periods (in some states, this action in and of itself constitutes child neglect). Their sense of community may lead them to lend their car to a neighbor or family member, even if the individual does not have a license. In a form of male bonding, a father may give his son a driving lesson before the son has obtained a proper learner's permit. In addition to learning how to read traffic signs in their new country, immigrant drivers should be educated about norms around cars and children.

## Misunderstandings with Schools

Falicov (1998) describes the entrance of the oldest child into school as the "first direct, sustained, and structured contact with an American institution" (p. 224) for many Latino families. This observation would also hold true for other immigrant groups. This contact presents numerous occasions for parents' behaviors to be interpreted as neglectful. Sometimes the seemingly neglectful practices result from poverty or circumstances that are difficult for a family to control, such as when children arrive late at school because of inadequate transportation, parents who work night shifts, or older children walking their younger siblings to school.

An immigrant family I know was reprimanded regularly over a period of months because of their failure to get their elementary-age children to school on time. Both parents worked two shifts, and simply could not wake up in time to give their children breakfast. Finally a compassionate counselor figured out a solution: the parents began waking up the children at 6:00 A.M., when they returned from their night shift and before they lay down to sleep, and put the children on the earlier high school bus. The children were able to eat a free breakfast at the high school, and then to walk down the block to their classes at the elementary school on time each day. Such a simple solution made by a conscientious counselor who took the time to think "outside the box" spared this family from further traumatic and punishing encounters with child protection services, and enabled the children to attend school appropriately and to eat breakfast each day.

School staff frequently characterize immigrant parents as uncaring because they miss parent–teacher conferences, not realizing that some of these parents are unable to read the notices or talk to the teacher in English. Moreover, schools often schedule these conferences at times that are inconvenient for working parents. (In 2004 the state legislature in South Carolina considered legislation to make it a felony for parents to miss three parent–teacher conferences in a row.) Immigrant parents sometimes avoid schools out of a sense of respect for the educators—they do not want to be seen as intruding upon a teacher's turf. Additionally, refugee and undocumented parents may fear walking into the school because of the official authority it represents. One Puerto Rican therapist noted the following:

> "Professionals have to get clear about who is the enemy. Or who is the client. [Professionals] have the client in front of them, but the client is responding to a totally unfair system, a totally unjust and ineffective system in the school: That because a kid is bilingual he's stupid. Or because he speaks two languages but doesn't speak English perfectly, he's stupid. . . . It's hard to hold onto hope when you have an oppressive system on top of you."

Immigrant parents are reprimanded for sending children to school when they are sick, even though they may have no reasonable alternative, and they may have been previously scolded for the child missing school. Also, less-educated parents are often made to feel inadequate if they cannot help their children with their homework. Bilingual children and their parents frequently feel alienated and ashamed at school, rather than applauded for having abilities in two or more languages.

Immigrant children may have substantial work obligations at home that interfere with their attendance and progress at school. These may include family responsibilities such as caring for siblings, cousins, or infirm grandparents, and employment such as helping out in the family business. The administrators of a school near me were puzzled by the frequent absences of three high-school-age Salvadoran "brothers." It turned out that the three boys were not brothers at all, but rather had been smuggled into the United States to drive a van and work in a furniture warehouse by an exploiter who provided them with housing and allowed them to attend school when they were not needed for work. These boys attended school rarely, performed poorly, and were frequently truant for almost a year before anyone in the school grew close enough to them to ascertain their true circumstances. They were part of the underground slave trade in immigrants that can be found throughout the United States and Canada (U.S. Department of State, 2004).

Parents from countries that have relatively easy transportation to and from the United States, such as Jamaica and Puerto Rico, may take their children out of school every winter for a month or two so that the children can celebrate Christmas and stay with members of their extended family during this time. This visit is more than a simple "vacation," it is a time to cement family and cultural bonds. For many parents, their children's contact with the "home country" is more central to their education than the weeks missed in school. Education authorities should give some thought about to the best way to handle this issue—whether it is better to provide children with schoolwork to bring with them, to give parents clear reasons why their children should not miss this time in school, or whether it is best to unenroll the children officially during their weeks away and re-enroll them upon their return—so the children will not have to be held back a grade for excessive absences.

## Medical Neglect

Dubowitz (1999) offers two criteria for establishing neglected healthcare: "(1) the lack of or delay in care involving actual or potential harm to the child's health and (2) the child not receiving the recommended care, which would offer a significant net benefit, outweighing the costs, side effects, and risks" (p. 121). Unfortunately, in practice these criteria are not always easy to determine.

Because explanations for physical ailments and ways to bring about cures vary so widely by culture, immigrant parents are sometimes vulnerable to charges of medical neglect. Immigrant parents are penalized for failing to immunize their children when they may not be able to afford preventive care or know how to access free immunization programs. In some cases, the children may indeed have been immunized but the parents do not have the paperwork to prove it because of a lack of continuity in healthcare.

Sometimes immigrant parents seek medical help for a child, but have trouble communicating about the child's condition (Erzinger, 1999). Professionals should explain how the healthcare system works, and help families gain access to quality healthcare. If a parent appears not to have attended to a child's medical condition, it is important to elicit the parents' explanation for the condition. The parent may believe that the child is cursed, has caught the evil eye, or is suffering from a draft or other traditional explanation of illness (Fadiman, 1997; Krajewski-Jaime, 1991).

Caring immigrant parents may avoid mainstream healthcare and opt for traditional medicine in the belief that this is the best way to heal their children or protect them from illness. In some cases these practices are helpful or indifferent, such as the use of most medicinal teas and herbs, acupuncture, or the laying on of hands. In other cases the traditional practices may lead to bruising and scarring, such as the Vietnamese practice of coining, or *cao gio*, and the Chinese *cheut sah*, in which a traditional medical practitioner or parent rubs the edge of a coin on or applies a hot spoon to a child's skin to relieve a variety of symptoms. Eastern European, Asian, and Mexican American families may practice cupping, in which hot cups are applied to parts of a child's body to create a vacuum that moves the blood to the surface of the body, creating bruises that are essentially large hickies. Russian, Asian, Arab, and African families sometimes practice moxibustion, in which incense or small balls of burning cotton, yarn, or herbs are applied to parts of the body, which may leave burns or scars. Somali Bantu families may rely on a traditional healer who will pray over the sick family member, and may heat up a metal rod or a piece of dry wood and then apply it to ailing body parts. While these cultural practices mimic abuse, the social science literature increasingly recommends that we show tolerance and respect for these practices because they were intended to preserve children's lives rather than to harm them (Levesque, 2001). Jurisdictions vary in how they handle these cases. In some cases, cultural evidence has been dismissed as a defense in court; in others, it has been used successfully to acquit or substantially reduce the charges against parents who acted in ways with their children that would customarily be considered abusive or neglectful (Levesque, 2001).

On the other hand, certain cultural healthcare practices have the potential to harm children permanently and must be stopped, regardless of the parents' intentions. For instance, some Central American parents give children potions containing mercury or use mercury to "clean" rooms of *el mal de ojo* (the evil eye), which is highly dangerous.

The inclusion of lead in folk remedies for various illnesses is disturbingly widespread, given that even minimal exposure to lead has been associated with serious neurological damage. Some Central American medications for *empacho* (a stomach ailment that may include vomiting, diarrhea, lethargy, and nausea) are almost pure lead. These medications include a bright orange powder that goes by the names of *azarcón, ruedo, corol, María Luísa, alarcón,* and *ligo;* a bright yellow powder called *greta;* and a white powder called *abayalde.* Other folk medicines containing high levels of lead include a red powder called *pay-loo-ah,* used by the Hmong for rash or fever; a brown powder called *ghasard,* a red powder called *kandu,* and a liquid called *bala goli,* used by Asian Indians for indigestion and stomach aches; kohl (also called *alkohl*), a powder used as eye makeup and also applied to skin infections and the navels of newborn children by some people from the Middle East; *farouk* and *santrinj,* used in some countries in the Middle East for teething; and *bint al zahab* and *al murrah,* used by some people from Saudi Arabia for colic (Texas Department of State Health Services, 2004; New South Wales Environmental Protection Agency, 2004).

Professionals who work with immigrants are well advised to ask them about the traditional remedies that they are using with their children. The remedies mentioned above and others may contain harmful levels of lead. You can get the folk remedies tested for the presence of lead, while at the same time informing the family of the risks of lead poisoning. Korbin (1999) advises us to honor the cultural importance of treating conditions such as *empacho*, while at the same time protecting children from high levels of toxins such as lead.

Most forms of genital cutting of girls, which is practiced by some African and Muslim families, are harmful. Practices range from partial removal of the clitoris to full removal of the external labia and clitoris and sewing the vagina shut. The more extreme of these practices can leave girls and women with difficulty passing their urine or menstrual blood, and make them highly vulnerable to infections including HIV/AIDS. Sometimes families from regions where female genital cutting is practiced will pool funds together to bring a person from their country of origin to perform this practice on their daughters in their new land (Hassan, 2004). In the United States and Canada, this is likely to be considered criminal assault. Many African families from regions where this genital cutting has been practiced have abandoned these customs, while others choose to nick the clitoris with a surgical tool and draw a drop or two of blood in a symbolic nod to cultural tradition.

Male circumcision (i.e., removing the foreskin of the penis) that is performed by a medical or trained religious professional is not considered a form of child abuse, perhaps because its practice is so widespread in Western culture. While male circumcision performed in early infancy has been found to be painful to the infant, this pain can be controlled through medication. Unlike most forms of female genital cutting, male circumcision does not result in long-term impairment of functioning.

To overcome their vulnerabilities to accusations of medical neglect, immigrant parents should be supplied by professionals with information about expectations and legal requirements in their communities regarding healthcare, and especially with information about free or low-cost healthcare. Professionals should also investigate their local healthcare providers' practices regarding sharing information with immigration authorities so that they can advise clients appropriately.

## Marriage by Capture and Forced Marriage of Minors

Issues concerning child sexual abuse and immigrant families are discussed extensively in Chapter 6. In this section I address issues that could be described as bride theft, marriage by capture, forced marriage, or simply "rape," depending on one's perspective and the circumstances.

In widely diverse cultures, a certain number of men have secured a wife through force. Although this custom is less widespread than it once was, it can still be found in some countries in Africa and Asia, in Kyrgyzstan and some of the other countries of the former Soviet Union, among the Hmong from Laos and some rural peoples of the Dominican Republic and Central America, and among some renegade Mormons in the United States.

Yang (2004) describes marriage by capture as "a continuing cultural practice among Hmong communities of America" (p. 38). This practice is just one of three ways the Hmong marry, the others being marriage by courtship (consensual) and marriage by elopement (when parents do not give permission for the marriage but both the bride and groom consent). In marriage by capture, a man kidnaps a young woman and rapes her. After holding her for 3 days, he arranges for a traditional Hmong go-between, called the *mej-koob*, to legitimize the marriage by arranging a bride price and performing a marriage ceremony. The girls are often between the ages of 14 and 18, whereas the men are typically between the ages of 18 and 30 (Yang, 2004). Sexual assault and rape are part of the marriage-by-capture custom. Although a young woman can reject her captor as a husband, her family is apt to pressure her to submit, since she has already engaged in sexual activity and only a marriage can save her and her family's reputation. Although marriage by capture is not the primary form of marriage among the Hmong in the United States, it still occurs. Authorities have responded with surprising leniency, often allowing Hmong men to use a cultural defense and plead guilty to charges that are substantially less severe than rape and kidnapping (Yang, 2004).

In rural parts of Central America and the Dominican Republic, there is a similar tradition of marriage by capture called *me robó* or *me llevó* ("he robbed me" or "he took me"). In some cases, a young woman will conspire with an older man, meet him in a designated spot, and the two of them will run off together. After a number of days she will contact her parents and report, "Me robó." The notion is that by presenting the initial pairing as against her will, she is preserving her honor. Now that her honor has been stained, her parents are forced to consider the two a legitimate couple and the two are considered married. A church wedding may even follow. In other cases, as among the Hmong, the young woman is in fact kidnapped. Sometimes, although the girl has given her consent, she may still be below the age of legal consent, and therefore the case may still be open for charges of rape, statutory rape, or child sexual abuse, as well as abduction of a minor. And finally, in some instances a man will trick a young woman or girl into spending some time with him and engaging in sexual activity. He pretends that this is meant to be an announcement of their engagement, and then will abandon her after having ruined her reputation.

In many cultures around the world, including some in Africa, Asia, and the Middle East, girls (and, less commonly, boys) may be forced into marriage by their parents. Arranged marriages differ from forced marriages. In arranged marriages, the families of both spouses take a leading role in making the arrangement, but both spouses can decide whether or not they wish to comply. In forced marriages, one or both of the spouses (usually the bride) are forced to comply against their will.

Families may persist in forcing their teenage children into marriage, even when they know it runs counter to the culture of their new homeland. They may be motivated by threats or promises, or believe that it is the most honorable way for marriages to be conducted, that they can secure citizenship or other benefits through the marriage, or that they can control their child's perceived sexual or other transgressions.

The British Association of Chief Police Officers (2000) released guidelines for the police on handling forced marriages, which are reported at the rate of about 200 per year in Britain but are thought to occur at a much higher rate. (I am not aware of a similar document in the United States or Canada.) The guidelines describe the motivations behind forced marriage and ways to handle it. The document asserts that there is usually criminal activity involved in forced marriage, including kidnapping, false imprisonment, harassment, assault, and rape. Guidelines include taking the victim's report seriously, maintaining confidentiality, and instructing the victim as to her rights. Sometimes the forced marriage has already occurred on foreign soil, sometimes it is planned to occur when the girl is forced on a trip overseas, and sometimes it occurs in the new country.

It can be extremely difficult for professionals to know how to handle situations of marriage-by-capture or forced marriage when members of the victim's cultural community claim these practices are acceptable in their country of origin. Yang (2004) makes a strong case that immigrant women and girls have the same right to protection from sexual assault and kidnapping as do native-born women. She writes that "the cultural defense fails to respect the victim's values and rights in America, and privileges the abductor's cultural standards. . . . Cultural preservation is important, but gender equality and justice are necessary for human rights" (p. 46). We must also remember that within every culture there are those who support and those who decry traditional practices, especially those practices in which certain people are victimized. People from all groups deserve protection from sexual assault and kidnapping.

## DOMESTIC VIOLENCE

Domestic violence, otherwise known as "wife beating" or "intimate partner violence," coexists with child abuse about half the time (Edleson, 1999). Husbands who beat their wives are much less likely to apply for permanent residence for their undocumented wives than husbands who do not beat their wives. Put plainly, immigration status appears to be another way in which abusive husbands control their wives. Abusive husbands often threaten their wives with deportation if they do not comply with the husband's wishes or if they threaten separation. Frequently, undocumented abused wives are afraid to cooperate with child protection authorities for fear that their husbands might retaliate by turning them in to immigration authorities. The *U Visa*, described below, offers undocumented women a measure of protection against this threat. Women who cooperate with investigations of child abuse and/or domestic violence have unusually good access to legal permanent residency, but are unlikely to be aware of this.

When intervening with a family with both domestic violence and child abuse that is from a culture different from one's own, it may be easy to accept explanations that this treatment of women is "cultural" and therefore not open to scrutiny or questioning by professionals. Fernando Mederos (2003) urges us to remember that there are "aspects of manhood in many cultures that support respectful and egalitarian relationships with women." He continues:

> I grew up in Cuba. My father was physically and psychologically abusive and embodied traditions of machismo in many ways. His first cousin is Jorge, a contemporary of my father's whom I have known for 50 years. Jorge is respectful and nurturing to his partner and family and is an egalitarian decision-maker. He is not violent, coercive or controlling. Jorge and my father were both imbedded in their culture as Cuban men. Jorge is not a feminist. He derived his sense of manhood from his milieu in Cuba in the 1930s onward, and he was somehow able to create a sense of manhood that, along with his positive characteristics, was also proud, assertive and fun-loving. In my culture, I see men who embody both of these polarities of manhood. When I established batterer intervention programs for Latinos in Boston in the 1990s, I saw something similar emerge amongst the men I worked with: many group participants realized that within their cultural traditions and life backgrounds they had clear choices and models of oppressive as well as nurturing and responsible manhood. This was crucial in their change process.

I am including this quote because it illustrates the variability within a single culture. Also, I have sometimes seen child abuse professionals assume that abusive practices are culturally based, and therefore hesitate to challenge them. Even when a certain behavior or attitude toward women or children does have a cultural underpinning, a culturally competent practitioner will work to increase safety for all family members, and demand accountability from abusive men (Almeida & Dolan-Delvecchio, 1999).

Battered immigrant women face several impediments to seeking protection and services, including language barriers, negative perceptions of the law enforcement and legal system, fear of deportation, cultural and religious issues, and discrimination (American Bar Association, 2001).

# BASIC U.S. IMMIGRATION DEFINITIONS

• *Immigrants* are also called "resident aliens." These are people who have been given permission to live indefinitely in the United States. In the first years of this millennium, a number of unprecedented laws were passed that restrict the rights of resident aliens and make them vulnerable to deportation.

• *Refugees or asylees* are people who have been granted asylum in the United States because they will be persecuted because of race, religion, national origin, political opinion, or membership in a social group if they are forced to return to their home country. A person granted asylum may reside in the United States until conditions are better for them to return. Individuals granted asylum may apply for permanent residence. Refugees have often undergone almost unimaginable hardships in their countries of origin, including torture, sexual assault, and being forced to witness the torture or murder of family members. In addition, escape from the country of origin may have been a harrowing process, including being forced to grant sexual favors in exchange for immigration papers, being hurt by pirates or bandits during the escape, being enslaved by military or rebel soldiers, starvation, illness, and the separation of families. Refugees often experience great fear and symptoms of posttraumatic stress.

• *Nonimmigrants* are people who have been granted permission to come to the United States for specific purposes and limited periods of time, such as students.

• *Undocumented aliens* are people who are living in the United States without official permission or whose permission has expired. This term is preferred over the term "illegal aliens," which implies that the person's entire being is illegal, or that the person has been engaged in criminal activity.

• *Naturalized citizens* are people who were born outside the United States but who have applied for and been granted citizenship in the United States.

• *U Visas* are available to immigrants who are either victims of—or who possess information concerning—a variety of criminal activities including ones that are most relevant to child abuse: rape, torture, incest, domestic violence, sexual assault, abusive sexual contact, prostitution, sexual exploitation, female genital mutilation, felonious assault, or solicitation to commit one of these offenses. A federal, state, or local official must certify that an investigation or prosecution would be harmed without the assistance of the immigrant or, in the case of a child, the immigrant's parent. Individuals granted U Visas may adjust to legal permanent resident status 3 years after they are granted the U Visa. Any immigrant who has information about child abuse, sexual assault, or domestic violence and who cooperates with an investigation may request a U Visa.

Whatever the results of the investigation, the immigrant's cooperation should entitle him or her to obtain this visa, paving the way to permanent residency.[1]

# SUGGESTIONS FOR IMPROVING CULTURAL COMPETENCE WITH IMMIGRANTS

## Gain Familiarity with the Culture

Learn about your area's immigrant cultures and history. Professionals who work closely with immigrants need to read books, attend cultural events, and make friends with members of immigrant communities. If your only contact with immigrant families is with your clients, who are usually in crisis, you will have a distorted view of their cultures. You should learn about the specific national origin and circumstance of immigration of the largest immigrant groups in your area, as well as facts about the specific families with whom you're working.

## Truth, Lies, and Immigration

As illustrated in the following example, getting basic demographic information from a refugee family or a family of recent immigrants may be especially difficult:

> A Liberian father who had been tortured and threatened with death fled to the U.S. embassy with several family members when civil war broke out in his country. His wife and their two children, along with his older sister and her two children, fled with him. They claimed that the older sister was his wife's mother and that her two children were their own. They could bring these extra three family members to the United States only by representing them as first-degree relatives in this way. They needed to lie to save their extended family. In the chaos of the war, they were able to obtain new documents and arrived safely in the United States as refugees.
>
> However, these are big secrets to keep. The children entered school, knowing they had a "grandma" who was really an aunt, "sis-

---

[1]For more information on the U Visa and other protections for immigrants in cases of domestic violence and child abuse, contact Legal Momentum's Immigrant Women Project in Washington, DC (*www.legalmomentum.org*), or the National Immigration Project of the National Lawyers Guild in Boston, Massachusetts (*www.nationalimmigrationproject.org*).

ters" who were really cousins, and so on. Their birthdays had also been falsified to make it all work out.

This family was called into the principal's office because the 8-year-old daughter was caught lying to her teacher. The family punished the girl for lying by placing a hot pepper on her tongue—they thought they were responding appropriately to what they interpreted as the school's request that they punish her. The child told a teacher about the punishment, and that teacher called in child protective services. The investigator working with the family had a hard time figuring out who was who and what had really happened. The family lied about basic demographic facts like birthdays and relationships. The lies looked suspicious, and the family appeared fearful, but not because they had anything to hide in the way of child abuse. Rather:

- They feared deportation for having lied upon entry.
- They feared losing their lease because they had so many people living in one apartment.
- They were afraid the niece and nephew—who they had said were their son and daughter—would lose health benefits because they would no longer qualify under the father's plan.
- They feared their children would be held back at school if their true ages were revealed.
- They were afraid of U.S. authorities because they were so mistreated by authorities in Liberia.

This was a loving, united family, which needed education about child-rearing norms in the United States, not punitive intervention. They needed reassurance that the social worker was not going to report them to immigration officials.

When working with immigrants, professionals sometimes notice that birth dates seem to keep shifting. Every time I escort my mother-in-law to the doctor so I can interpret for her and I ask her birth date, she says, "Which one?" She was born in a small town in Portugal where there was a law mandating that parents register their children within a couple of months of the child's birth. Because her parents were poor and lived far from the registry office, and because they did not want to attract "the evil eye" by taking her survival for granted before passing those crucial first months of life, her parents waited several months before registering her. To conform to the law, they had to say she was just 2 months old. Hence, she has two birthdays: an official one that is on all her documents, and her real date of birth, which the family celebrates. This kind of situation is not uncommon with immigrant families.

Chinese families often celebrate the day a person was conceived, rather than the day the person was born, as the birthday. There may also be confusion when translating dates from the Chinese to the Western calendar. Somali Bantus and people from other traditional agricultural societies often do not keep track of birth dates or celebrate birthdays. Children's maturity is traditionally measured by how grown up they look and what they are able to do, rather than by a chronological date.

Other immigrants create new stories including new dates to hide incidents that they consider shameful—such as a pregnancy resulting from a rape, children born out of wedlock, and even previous marriages or liaisons. People who come from rural societies or those whose lives have been disrupted by war or natural disaster may simply have no idea of their "true" birthday on a Western calendar.

Fleeing war or persecution, immigrants are often faced with situations where they have to find "the right story" so they can obtain refugee status. They may believe that they need to present in one way to obtain entrance into refugee camps, to present another story to gain entrance into the United States or Canada, and to frame their situation in a third way to be granted official refugee status. Rumors abound in refugee camps about what is an "acceptable" story to the authorities, and families with legitimate claims to refugee status sometimes distort their histories in response to these rumors. If their lies are discovered, the family is likely to face deportation, regardless of the true dangers they face if deported.

Children from families of all kinds are raised to tell lies: to hide immigration status or an illegal activity, to keep secret a birthday surprise, or to get the kids-price meal at a restaurant. While lying may be of concern to professionals and certainly complicates matters, it does not necessarily indicate that child abuse has occurred.

How should professionals handle concerns about truthfulness with immigrant families? It is important to gain the family's trust, clarify the professional role, and let the family know who will have access to the information they provide. We should acknowledge that in the process of immigration many families have had to tell new stories about their lives. We should ask for the truth *about things that matter*, but avoid punishing or embarrassing immigrant parents who lie about unimportant or unrelated matters. So, for instance, an investigator could say to a family:

"I'm having trouble understanding certain things here. There may be things you are afraid to tell me, or don't want to talk about in front of the children. I don't need to know everything today. But I would like to meet alone with the parents now to help me understand those things that *are* important for me to understand today."

By speaking with the parents alone, without children present, the professional allows the parents to save face.

In democracies we say "The truth will make you free." In Spanish there is a saying, "*La verdad no mata, pero incomoda*" (Truth doesn't kill, but it makes us uncomfortable). In fact, truth *can* kill people living under repressive governments. Telling stories that are not entirely truthful may have helped certain immigrants and refugees to survive—a reality that is alien to most people growing up in the United States and Canada. Lying for self-protection is a hard habit to break. Child abuse professionals need to seek the truth, but should do it sensitively after establishing trust and without humiliating their clients.

When working with people of uncertain immigration status, it is always helpful to be able to say, "Our agency has a policy—we do not release information to immigration authorities." If your agency does not have such a policy, it should develop one—and this should be posted in several languages in the waiting room and in written materials. In some jurisdictions, however, law enforcement and child protective services may be required to report certain classes of crimes committed by undocumented people to the U.S. Immigration and Naturalization Service. You should become aware of your responsibilities in this regard.

## Be Helpful as Soon as Possible

Many immigrant families are unfamiliar with social services and do not expect that interventions will help. The professional's reputation and working relationship will be established in the first meeting. One social worker from Colombia shared her approach:

> "I start with the presenting problem, and I work with behavioral things that the parents can do to help the child. I work on the rules in the house and the boundaries in the family. And I connect with the father, even if he refuses to meet with me in the beginning. I try to make him feel his importance, and I get in with the family through him."

Doing something concrete that is helpful to a family, such as translating a letter from a landlord, making a call to a teacher, arranging for daycare or fuel vouchers, enrolling a parent in English lessons, contacting a soup kitchen, or putting the family in contact with a medical provider can make for the beginning of a trusting relationship. Immigrant families who are less acculturated need support of all kinds. The abstract, more long-term "help" that social service providers often give may be less valued, immediately, than something a family can put their hands on or eat that very night. Once the immigrant family trusts that the provider means well and can deliver, they are likely to be immensely loyal.

## Demonstrate Caring, Warmth, and Respect

Immigrants often describe U.S. and Canadian professionals as cold and distant. To work effectively, professionals should be warm and demonstrate caring. The professional should show the client a personal and specific caring for him or her (*personalismo* in Spanish), not simply generalized empathy. This can be achieved by remembering details about the client's situation, starting meetings with time to socialize, and truly listening to the client's concerns.

Because of their experiences with discrimination, many immigrants who are involved with the social service system are acutely sensitive—maybe even overly sensitive—to possible demonstrations of disrespect. For instance, many professionals like to dress informally in jeans and sneakers. An immigrant adult may be so insulted by this perceived lack of professionalism and respect that he or she will not return for a second appointment. It may appear to the immigrant client that the professional who has "dressed down" is not taking his or her job seriously.

One Puerto Rican client I interviewed suggested that professionals communicate the following:

> "I'm not here to judge you. I am not God. I am just a human being, just like you are. Whatever you've gone through, I'm here to help. And I'll let you know if I can help and I'll let you know if I can't help, but we'll try. And if we both work at it, we're going to get some place. . . . We have to both be together and be honest with each other, not try to pull one over on the other."

## Be Careful in Your Use of Time

Although most professionals are constrained by heavy caseloads, managed care, and busy schedules, it is important to pay attention to how we handle time with our immigrant clients. Time spent building the relationship is not wasted but rather is essential to the success of our work. To accommodate this need many professionals schedule longer sessions with their immigrant clients, particularly early in the course of their work together. Professionals often grow frustrated with immigrant clients who arrive at scheduled meetings late—sometimes hours late. It is important to explore this issue with the clients rather than making threats such as "Two more missed sessions and I can't see you anymore" or "If you are not on time for our appointments, I have to tell your social worker that you are noncompliant." The client may be late because the appointments are not scheduled at a convenient time, but the client does not realize he or she can request a different time, or does not want to inconvenience the professional by requesting a different time. Sometimes clients are late because they cannot afford the transportation or childcare that would enable them to attend appointments punctually. Sometimes clients are late because of experiences in their countries of origin and their new countries where they have to spend hours and hours in waiting rooms to meet with a doctor. Sometimes they simply have a different sense of what a starting time means. Vietnamese clients will often arrive late so as not to appear overly enthusiastic. I experienced a culturally different sense of time once with a Nigerian student, who arrived at class consistently 15 or 20 minutes after it had begun. After a number of class sessions I finally asked him if something specific was interfering with his arriving at class on time. He replied, "Oh, would you like me to be here from the beginning?" He was never late again. Clear communication is key.

Professionals should be especially careful to avoid rushing their immigrant clients, if at all possible. This rushing, which is so characteristic of Western society, may be interpreted as evidence of a lack of caring and respect.

## Language Preference

When working with an immigrant family, it is important to ask about the language(s) they prefer to speak, and their educational backgrounds. Some immigrants are highly educated, some are illiterate, but most fall in between. Professionals should not assume that the immigrants they work with have low levels of education or intelligence simply because they do not speak English fluently.

Rich information can often be obtained by asking about the language(s) a family speaks. It may turn out that the father is from one ethnic group and speaks one language with his children, while the mother speaks another, and the entire family has learned to speak a third language that was used in public settings in their country of origin.

Sometimes a family will deny that it needs an interpreter, overlooking the fact that a key family member, such as the mother, may not speak English. They may be so accustomed to leaving the mother out of conversations, or having a child interpret for the mother, that they do not even see the ways in which using an interpreter could enhance their work with professionals.

Being allowed to speak in one's first language, "the language of the heart," can allow a person's personality to shine forth in a way that may be impossible while speaking a second language. For instance, a Brazilian mother may seem removed, disinterested, formal, and cold in English, but she may brighten considerably and interact in a lively way with her children when speaking Portuguese. If she uses her English mostly in formal interactions with her host culture, which she may experience as frightening, an assessment conducted solely in English will not tap into her true knowledge, ability, and personality. (See Chapter 1 for further discussion of language.) The author and poet Julia Alvarez (2004) writes of the alienation of speaking in a second language: "I didn't know if I could ever show genuine feeling in a borrowed tongue" (p. 29).

## Language Competency as a Legal Obligation

Title VI of the Civil Rights Act of 1964 forbids discrimination against any person on the basis of national origin in offering any services that receive federal financial assistance. This has been interpreted by the courts to include delivering adequate services to any individual who does not understand English, including arranging for interpreters, as well as informing clients or patients that interpreters are available. On August 11, 2000, President Clinton signed an executive order stating that all agencies receiving federal assistance must provide services that are accessible to people with limited English proficiency. These stipulations apply to most healthcare, legal, criminal justice, education, and social welfare settings. Besides the moral obligation to provide these services, agencies should be advised that they ignore these legal obligations at their own peril.

Immigrants deserve prompt access to high-quality interpreters: this is the law. Prohibited practices include services that are more limited in scope or of a lower quality; unreasonable delays; limited participation in a program or activity; failure to inform people with limited English proficiency (LEP) of their right to an interpreter; and requiring people to provide their own interpreters (see the U.S. Department of Justice websites for further information on obligations toward people with limited English proficiency). Because this is a federal obligation, it is in force even in states with "English only" laws. (For more information, see Chapter 7.)

## Translated Documents

The problems for immigrant families in the child welfare system are exacerbated by a serious shortage of translated material at government and private agencies (see Chapter 7). I have conducted trainings in a large northeastern city where 40% of the school population was Latino, but *none* of the current child protective services documents were available in Spanish. The workers told me they had some old handouts in Spanish, but these did not elaborate on important changes that had been instituted 4 years earlier.

Every day families were being asked to sign forms, including treatment plans, that they could not understand, and then children were permanently removed from their homes when these families failed to comply. Although the state agency serving this major city had been informed of the need to translate documents, and had apparently translated a limited number of forms a decade earlier, the new, computer-ready forms had not been translated. Unfortunately, this problem is common throughout the country, and is even more drastic for families who speak languages that are less widespread than Spanish.

Even qualified bilingual social workers have described their frustration when they must ask families to sign legal documents that the families do not understand. The bilingual workers do their best to translate documents spontaneously at the moment, but the immigrant families have no chance to study them, to think about possible consequences, or to show the documents to trusted friends for advice. This kind of situation is far worse if the social worker does not speak the clients' language fluently. Some immigrant groups, such as Cambodians, Russians, and the Hmong, very rarely have the opportunity to work with professionals who speak their language, virtually guaranteeing that the services they receive will be inferior to those received by native speakers of English.

Paperwork must be available in all the languages of the clients in our communities. Providing an interpreter to help with filling out forms, one client at a time, is time-consuming and expensive. (However, providing an interpreter is still more effective than expecting nonnative speakers of English to fend for themselves.) Clients who have an opportunity to fill out paperwork in their own languages are apt to feel more empowered and welcomed than clients who have to seek others' help with basic paperwork. Often, several state or local agencies find it advantageous to develop uniform intake forms, for instance, and then pool their resources for translating these into a variety of languages. Much of the work that I have seen in child maltreatment that has been translated into Spanish or Portuguese— intake forms, research surveys, flyers, even signs on buildings—has been poorly translated and is nearly incomprehensible to native speakers.

Occasionally, paperwork has been translated into a variety of languages, but no qualified professional has checked it over to assess the quality of the translation. For instance, in an attempt to reach out to the diverse immigrant communities in my area, the local middle school recently printed in the school newspaper a short announcement in a variety of languages that the school would make translators available to help parents read the newsletter or any other school communications. While this was certainly done with the best of intentions, the paragraphs in Portuguese and Spanish were unintelligible (I cannot comment on the paragraphs in Tibetan, Khmer, and Mandarin). The principal had relied on children within the school to translate these paragraphs from English. While it is possible that these children *speak* their first language fluently, it was clear that their written skills were poor. The paragraphs were full of spelling and grammatical errors, and even an invented word or two, adapted from English. If Spanish or Portuguese speakers were to read these paragraphs, they would have trouble understanding them, and would certainly doubt the school's commitment to reaching nonnative speakers of English. Translations of official documents must be done by people who are fluent *writers* of the language in question. Presenting immigrant families with materials full of errors is just as egregious as presenting English-speaking families with materials full of errors—it damages the school's or agency's credibility.

I have attended meetings at schools, hospitals, and mental health clinics where the professionals stated that certain forms were available in languages other than English, but had neglected to bring these along for the meeting. Translated materials must be easily available to those who need them, whenever they might be needed.

## CONCLUDING THOUGHTS

In the United States and Canada, most professionals hold a highly individualistic view of child maltreatment (Fontes, 1995a). That is, they look upon maltreatment as something that parents inflict on children. They view issues of child poverty and hunger, inadequate housing and healthcare, child prostitution, overcrowded and underfunded schools, and dangerous neighborhoods as something other than child maltreatment. This delimiting of the category of "child maltreatment" does not hold in most other nations, where concerns about human rights and children's basic human needs dominate the discourse (Finkelhor & Korbin, 1988). Before focusing on possible family dysfunction, professionals would be well advised to consider the interactive effects of social stress, individual psychology, poverty, and culture on child maltreatment (Zayas, 1992). Certainly, improving the material and social conditions of immigrant families will not only benefit children directly, it will also make parenting easier and less stressful. Therefore, professionals who care about the well-being of their immigrant clients would be well advised to work to bring about changes on a systemic level.

Helping parents cope with their economic and social stress is apt to improve parenting and reduce levels of neglect and physical abuse. Professionals may need to intervene in ways that stretch their traditional roles, through political activism (e.g., petitioning civil authorities for better legal protections for immigrants), advocacy (e.g., helping parents manage their relationships with social services), and counseling on immigration issues (e.g., helping families understand how their differing levels of acculturation affect them). When working with immigrant families we should try to address the family's welfare in general rather than just the narrowest questions of child abuse.

Immigrant families caught in the child welfare system often fail to comprehend the system that has taken over their lives—such a system may not exist in their home countries. In much of the world, only the most extreme cases of child abuse will receive intervention, and this may consist of removing the children to an orphanage, or of the local people beating up a sexual offender. In Spanish, for instance, there is no exact word or concept for "foster family," "foster care," "foster mother," "preadoptive home," "parenting class," or many of the other concepts that are so central to our work. Similarly, in the Russian language there is no term for "battering," "batterers," or "battered woman."

Immigrant children deserve the same protection from child abuse as all other children, and this includes formulating and implementing responses that take into account the immigrants' special needs. Psychoeducation that includes detailed information about cultural expectations for child rearing in the United States—geared especially for immigrant families—would seem to be a key part of any child abuse intervention or prevention program involving immigrant families.

These generalizations about working with immigrant families are meant to be suggestive rather than exhaustive. To work well with clients from diverse cultures, professionals must approach cultural issues with the same seriousness as they approach other issues of professional development. They must seek to understand the ecosystem in which the clients live. Only then will every child and family affected by child maltreatment receive the high-quality professional response they deserve.

## QUESTIONS TO THINK ABOUT AND DISCUSS

1. How might the process of immigration change the way a family raises its children?

2. What are the origins of the main immigrant groups in your area, and what does your agency need to do to meet their needs better?

3. What are some of your assumptions about immigrant families, or about families from a particular immigrant group?

4. What are some of the ways you can demonstrate your respect toward a parent from an immigrant family?

5. If you were going to explain to a group of immigrant parents what they needed to know to raise their children in your country, what are some of the main points you would make?

CHAPTER THREE

# Assessing Diverse Families for Child Maltreatment

There is no inherent contradiction between
incorporating culture in child protection and ensuring
child well-being. It does not follow that if cultural
diversity is accommodated in child protection efforts,
differing standards for different cultures will emerge
and children will suffer as a result.
—KORBIN AND SPILSBURY (1999, p. 69)

This chapter provides information on how to reduce bias when assessing
for child maltreatment among culturally diverse families. It describes some
of the ways child abuse professionals commonly mistake cultural differences for child abuse or overlook child abuse in families that differ from
them culturally. It also discusses the utility of formal risk assessment instruments and structured decision making when assessing culturally
diverse families.

Discussing assessment raises a particularly urgent and contentious issue: ethnic and racial differences in ushering families into the child welfare
system. While national incidence studies indicate that there are *no significant differences in maltreatment rates* between African Americans and
Whites (National Center on Child Abuse and Neglect, 1996), for instance,
"in most jurisdictions African Americans are more likely than Whites, His-
panics or Asians to have allegations of maltreatment substantiated and to
have children placed in out-of-home care" (Baird, Ereth, & Wagner, 1999,
p. 3). Fairness and accuracy in the assessment of maltreatment is clearly an
urgent priority.

On the level of the individual professional, common questions when
thinking about assessing risk to a child include:

- "Do I have enough suspicion to file a report?"
- "Is the evidence strong enough to substantiate or support a report that child maltreatment has occurred or a child is at risk?"
- "Is the family safe enough for the child to remain in the home or to be reunited with his or her family?"
- "Can safety be achieved through support rather than placement?"

This chapter is directed to mandated reporters who are trying to decide whether a behavior they have witnessed or heard about constitutes a "reasonable suspicion" and therefore needs to be reported (the exact wording varies by state). It is also directed to child protection investigators who may be faced with deciding whether to "substantiate" or "support" a report of child maltreatment. And it is directed to people who work in the legal and child welfare systems, such as social workers, attorneys, judges, and guardians ad litem, who are considering abusive behaviors that have occurred and who are trying to decide how to weigh these behaviors in determining the best placement for a child. These various professionals differ in their responsibilities, but all of them may get caught up in the same issues involving cultural differences. Information relevant to assessment is also contained in other chapters in this book, particularly Chapters 2, 4, and 5, which focus on working with immigrants, interviewing, and physical discipline and abuse, respectively.

In this chapter I address ways to overcome some of the challenges that confront professionals in making the above determinations when the family under consideration is from a minority cultural group. My intention in this chapter is to help professionals avoid bias in their decision-making process—whether that bias is for or against members of a particular group. I am *not* assuming that the professionals are from the dominant group. Regardless of their own cultural background, most professionals in North America have been schooled to see people from the dominant group as the norm and people from other groups as deviant (see Chapter 1).

Assessing child abuse is like trying to keep your balance on a seesaw. If you lean too much in one direction, you are in danger of disrupting family life unnecessarily to "protect" children who do not actually need the intervention. If you lean too much in the other direction, you may fail to protect children who are in dangerous situations. In less severe circumstances, a faulty assessment may lead to a mismatch between services and client needs. In the most severe circumstances, a safe family may be permanently torn apart or a child may end up dead because of an incorrect assessment of the dangers. When there are cultural differences between the professionals and the families involved, it can be especially tricky to maintain equilibrium and provide quality services. In this chapter I examine the difficult questions of how to assess for child maltreatment when there are cultural differences between the professional, on the one hand, and the child and his or her family, on the other. The more we know about the family's culture, the less likely we are to err in either direction.

## WHAT CONSTITUTES A SUSPICION, AND WHAT'S CULTURE GOT TO DO WITH IT?

Most professionals experience a great deal of ambivalence about how and when they should follow up on their suspicions of child abuse by contacting child protective services or the police. We worry that our reports will drive families away, and that children will be "lost" in this way. Despite our own and our colleagues' best intentions, many of us have seen protective service interventions that inflicted harm rather than provided help. Where there is a racial, ethnic, or religious difference between the provider and the child, professionals may also fear that they will be perceived as discriminatory if they file a report. They may be concerned that they lack the necessary cultural information to distinguish between abuse and unfamiliar child-rearing practices.

Mandated reporters are obligated to report suspected maltreatment when they encounter it while they are carrying out their professional duties. In most states, people who work regularly with children are considered mandated reporters (ranging from school bus drivers to teachers, barbers, and psychotherapists). In Indiana, *all* adults are considered mandated reporters. The legal language varies slightly from state to state, but most states require that a report be made to the police or child protective services when there is "cause to believe" or "reasonable cause to believe" that a child is at risk for maltreatment or that such maltreatment is occurring or may have occurred (Zellman & Fair, 2002). The suspicion should be "reasonable" based on the professional's training and experience. The mandated reporter is required to make a report within a specified period. Reporters are not required to investigate or to be certain that the abuse has occurred. In fact, well-meaning but poorly trained mandated reporters who make a lot of inquiries while trying to begin the investigation themselves may put a child or a legal case at serious risk.

Research points to racial *and* economic bias on the part of mandated reporters (Charlow, 2001–2002; Roberts, 2002). That is, mandated reporters appear to be more likely to suspect and report child abuse if the injury is sustained by a child from a poor family or a Black or Native American family. In addition, Black, Latino, and Native American families are far more likely to be poor than White families, thus increasing the likelihood that they will be suspected and reported for child maltreatment on two counts—ethnicity *and* poverty. It may be that professionals are more apt to screen for and then report child abuse in minority families because their biases lead them to suspect substandard parenting or to confuse cultural practices with substandard parenting (see Chipungu & Bent-Goodley, 2003).

Some researchers assert that the problem of racial disproportionality in child welfare does not derive from reporting biases but rather from the poverty in which African American, Native American, and Latino children live, as compared to White and Asian American children. For example, neglect is more likely to be found among the poor. Therefore, members of ethnic groups who are more often poor are more frequently reported for neglect (Charlow, 2001–2003; Myers, 2003). Roberts (2000) rejects this argument, however, pointing out that if the issue was purely economic, Latino children would be reported and removed from their homes at rates similar to Black children, and this is simply not the case.

Specific contexts may determine whether someone is overly likely or overly hesitant to report a suspicion. In his study of teachers' reporting practices in schools, Ron Wilson (personal communication, 1999) found that teachers regularly overlooked clear evidence of neglect and abuse presented by African American children in poor neighborhoods. This was true for both White and Black teachers, but more common for White teachers. He hypothesized that the White teachers were hesitant to report for three main reasons:

1. They had grown accustomed to the high levels of poverty in the neighborhood and failed to notice when children were neglected.
2. They were afraid of being perceived as racist.
3. They felt genuinely confused about child discipline techniques that appeared to have a cultural foundation but apparently crossed the line into abuse.

Because they differed from the children they were teaching in terms of race, culture, and social class, the White teachers overlooked signs of "reportable" problems such as children regularly complaining that they were hungry, describing beatings, or showing bruises.

Professionals should remember that children from all cultural groups can be vulnerable to child abuse and neglect, and that all children deserve the same level of protection and safety. Therefore, it behooves us to report suspicions of abuse and neglect impacting all children, regardless of their cultural background (Fontes, 2000). Immigrant, minority, and low-income families are apt to be less familiar with the potential benefits of social services and may view them with caution or downright suspicion. However, this should not cause us to neglect our legal (and moral) obligation to report suspected child abuse and neglect. The important goal is to make sure that the reporting and interventions are conducted in culturally competent ways (see Fontes, 1995a).

That said, it might be hard for people from one culture to tell whether behaviors among people from a different culture justify suspicions of child abuse. To compound this problem, White teachers, guidance counselors, and neighbors sometimes report that they are less likely to approach a parent from a different culture with concerns about a child (such as poor hygiene or misbehavior) because they fear that they may be misunderstood and accused of prejudice. But this kind of discussion should not be avoided. Often the discussion alone allays suspicions and sets the stage for a helpful intervention. For instance:

> A kindergarten teacher noticed that unlike the other Black children in her class, who arrived at school well dressed each day, Regina arrived with unkempt hair. Also, although Regina was always clean and her clothes were neat, she wore flip-flops and a light dress despite the cool weather. Regina did not speak much. The teacher arranged to meet the child's mother, who revealed to her that the family had recently emigrated from Jamaica, that they had a very limited income, that the mother was allowing her daughter's hair to form dreadlocks, and that the family had not yet purchased winter clothes. The mother also confided that although Regina spoke freely at home, she was too nervous to speak at school because she was afraid the other children would tease her about her Jamaican accent and vocabulary. The mother gratefully accepted the teacher's offer to "round up" some winter clothes for her family, which the teacher sent home discreetly one day, along with a list of community resources that might interest the family. The teacher then made a special effort to facilitate Regina's friendships with other girls in the class. The teacher made international diversity a focus of the curriculum for several days, which gave Regina a kind of "star" status in the classroom. Regina continued to wear dreadlocks, which she tied up occasionally in a colorful scarf.

Because Regina seemed essentially well cared for, the teacher decided to contact the parents first, and obviated the need to initiate a report of suspected neglect. This turned out to be an ideal decision all around.

On the other hand, mandated reporters should not fail to report reasonable suspicion of abuse simply because of a cultural difference. For example, while playing the Talking, Feeling, and Doing Game (Gardner, 1973) with his school counselor one day, 6-year-old Vothy, whose family was from Cambodia, burst into tears when he picked a card that told him to say something he didn't like about his father. He said that his father would beat him if he did this, and he lifted up his shirt to show marks that he said were from a previous beating. The counselor did not know if—in fact—the marks were caused by a beating or by a Cambodian healing practice such as coining. Because Vothy said they were caused by a beating, the counselor appropriately called child protective services, which launched an investigation.

In sum, in walking that tightrope between taking the leap to report or not to report, and risk over- or underreacting, we must make sure we protect all children. At the same time, we must also make sure our biases for or against members of a certain group, or any discomfort we might feel with members of a certain group, do not make us either too eager or too hesitant to report. If a behavior raises concern, we can discuss the concern with a cultural informant while protecting privacy, discuss the concern with a colleague, or screen the issue with protective services anonymously before making our decision. However, if a concern is a suspicion, it must be reported.

## IS IT MALTREATMENT? IS THE CHILD AT RISK?

Child abuse is defined in slightly different ways in different state statutes. But the definition usually includes the concepts of harm, injury, or impairment, or risk of these problems. Determining whether a given act constitutes child maltreatment may seem like a straightforward process, but often it is not. How much harm is too much? It can be argued that when a child is given a breakfast cereal she doesn't like one morning, and therefore doesn't eat breakfast and is hungry in school until lunch, the child has been harmed. However, few would argue that this situation constitutes child neglect unless it occurs repeatedly. Exposure to many hours of television has been found to harm children's cognitive achievement and contribute to obesity, and yet few would argue that caretakers who allow their children to watch many hours of television are abusive. And how much risk is too much? Every year many children are severely injured and some die in football accidents, and yet few would argue that parents who allow their children to participate in contact sports are exposing them to abusive levels of risk. If a kindergartener breaks his arm while playing unsupervised in a stairwell, his parents may be subject to sanctions for neglect. However, if the same parents allow their child to ski and he breaks his arm, this is not considered neglectful. Clearly, cultural norms shape how we evaluate abuse and risk.

In many agencies, the concept informally cited for judging whether a punishment constitutes physical abuse is "leaving a mark." But even this concept is open to interpretation. If a mark lasts only a few moments, does that constitute a "mark?" What if it lasts 1 hour? What if it lasts 6 hours? If an adult twists a child's arm up behind his back so that it aches but leaves no sign of a bruise, is that child abuse? Does our decision depend on how long the arm is sore? Often, I'm afraid, assessments of "harm" and "risk" hinge on "soft" factors such as how articulate the parent might be and how comfortable the worker is with the parent, rather than on an objective evaluation of facts. (See the section of this chapter on assessment instruments, below.)

Even though I cannot address all possible dilemmas that might arise, I would like to discuss some of the most common issues that might compli- cate the assessment process when we work with immigrant and ethnic mi- nority families. The next sections address "false positives," cases in which workers substantiate child abuse where none exists, and "false negatives," where workers fail to substantiate child maltreatment—in both cases because of cultural issues.

## False Positives: "Finding" Abuse That Is Not Present

False positives in child welfare often result from ethnocentrism, where the professional sees his or her own beliefs and practices as superior, and mis- identifies differing cultural practices as maltreatment (Korbin & Spilsbury, 1999). When ethnocentrism prevails, the beliefs and behaviors of the dominant culture are imposed on other populations, and nonmainstream childcare practices are mistakenly viewed as pathological even when there is no harm to children.

## Sleeping Arrangements

Some families from traditional peasant cultures in Asia, Africa, and South America are incorrectly substantiated for neglect because their children sleep on the floor (Ivy Duong, private communication, May 2003). Before substantiating such a claim it would be important to determine whether this practice is traditional in the family's country of origin, whether the parents also sleep on the floor, and whether the sleeping space on the floor is clean and sanitary. Some Asian families use clean and comfortable mats for sleeping on the floor that they roll up each morning, leaving investiga- tors scratching their heads as they search for beds.

Families may be incorrectly found to be negligent or suspected of sexual abuse because they share beds, when sharing a bed may be cus- tomary in their country of origin and should not be seen in and of itself as being indicative of sexual abuse (Falicov, 1998). In some countries, such as Korea, it is traditional for the mother to sleep with her children in a room separate from the father who sleeps alone. (However, of course, even if sharing a bed or a hammock may be customary, sexual abuse *still* could be occurring.) Additionally, while it is common for children in families who share close quarters to be exposed to the sounds of their parents' lovemaking, this exposure might still be experienced by the child as uncomfortable and even abusive (Fontes, Cruz, & Tabachnick, 2001).

Co-sleeping itself may be problematic when children are beginning to mature physically and become aware of sexual urges, or if the adults have poor boundaries. Under normal circumstances, co-sleeping of nursing mothers with their infants facilitates nursing and the mother–child bond and should not be seen as problematic. Indeed, such co-sleeping may enhance the mother's ability to nurse and meet her child's needs.

Co-sleeping of infants with siblings or with adults may pose other risks, however. Research suggests co-sleeping may contribute to deaths from sudden infant death syndrome (SIDS), particularly when the bedding is soft, when children are placed face-down, and when they are sleeping on something other than a bed (e.g., a sofa). The ratio of Black to White deaths from SIDS is more than two to one. Economic factors appear to contribute, since some families cannot afford a bed for everyone in the household, including a crib that is appropriate for infants. A study by Hauck et al. (2003) recommends that parents and other caretakers should learn to place infants on their backs to sleep, should use firm bedding and avoid pillows, and avoid co-sleeping, especially on a sofa. Co-sleeping is problematic when the person (or people) in bed with the infant is obese, is impaired by drug or alcohol abuse, or is not the child's parent. It may be worth noting that in countries where co-sleeping is common, bedding is typically firmer, flatter, and has less excess covering such as blankets and pillows, and therefore poses less of a risk of SIDS and infant suffocation than the bedding used in Western countries.

In most of the world's cultures children sleep in the same bed or at least the same room as their parents. People from cultures as diverse as the Maya of Mexico, the Iu Mien of Southeast Asia, and different groups in East Africa respond in horror when they hear that children in the United States and Canada are often expected to sleep in a room alone, either from birth or from a very young age (Rogoff, 2003). Except for the situations of young infants discussed above, it would seem callous and ethnocentric for professionals to interfere with a family's culturally based sleeping practices if no problem has been noted with the current arrangements. If an investigation is conducted and there are other indicators of problems, or if the children are expressing a desire to sleep separately, or if the children are beyond preschool age, professionals should discuss with caretakers the advantages of some independence at night for their children.

## Flexible Boundaries

Unlike middle-class and upper-middle-class persons from the dominant cultural groups, people with a low income and people from many immigrant groups often have fluid boundaries around their selves and around their household. In describing Latino families, Falicov (1998) has referred to this as the *familial self*, "a sense of self that includes one's close relationships as part of who one is" (p. 163). Roland (1994) has also used the term "familial self" to describe Japanese and Indian people. When people have this extended sense of self, they may be more apt to share their homes, money, clothing, and even beds with relatives and family friends. It can become virtually impossible to close the door to a relative who needs a place to stay or who has decided to make an extended visit. A nuclear family that has saved assiduously to change apartments or send their child to college may inexplicably (or so it seems to someone from the outside) give their savings to a relative who needs medical care, a funeral, or a ticket from their home country. Among traditional families, this sharing of resources is not subject to debate; it is just what one does.

Sharing resources in this way creates a wider safety net than that provided by the societal institutions at large, thereby enabling families that may be stressed or near the poverty line to survive. Families may share meals, child- or elder care, transportation, and other resources. However, the fluidity of household boundaries can create dilemmas for the investigator who has learned to view the presence of adults other than parents as a risk factor. For example, perhaps a foster family has promised not to allow anyone who has not been approved to stay in the home, but at the next visit the investigator finds some new people—maybe even an entire family—in the household. Tío (Uncle) Pedro may have called over the weekend, saying his air conditioning was broken and he needed a cool place to stay, and there was simply no way to refuse him. To refuse to take him in, or to say that he could not come until he had been "approved" by a social service agency, would be an unimaginable insult. Even if Tío Pedro has some kind of criminal record, the family may not feel at liberty to turn him away. The family may be slow to grasp that they may lose their foster care license for such an infraction. In many societies, including, sometimes, the United States and Canada, a seemingly minor infraction of this kind can be "worked out" to everyone's satisfaction if there is goodwill on the part of the authorities in power and an empathic connection between the authority and the family.

Another example: A Korean family may give an investigator full information about who "lives" in the home, but neglect to mention that every weekend a cousin's family from the next city stays with them so they can attend their Korean-language church services together on Sunday.

Household compositions may not be as fixed as they are in families from the dominant cultural group, and this may seem so ordinary to the family that they neglect even to mention it.

The issue of fluid household composition might emerge in a different way. A family may hesitate to tell investigators the full truth about who lives in their home. They might describe their nuclear family only, knowing that this is the norm in their new country. Only after trust has been built will they reveal that an additional family shares the apartment, or that friends or even renters are sleeping in the kids' room and that the kids are all sharing a bed in another room.

How should an investigator handle these issues? If a family has failed to reveal the full truth or has lied, it would be important to try to find out the nature of the misrepresentation and the motivation behind it before approaching the family too harshly. Maybe they did not want to tell the investigator about every person who lives in the home because they have exceeded the limit allowed by their lease, or because the guest is undocumented, or because the additional person has a disability and is therefore stigmatized—not for any more nefarious reason. If the additional person or people who are staying in the home have been determined to put the child at risk, or if the loose boundaries around the household seem to be a problem (e.g., prostitution or drug dealing are bringing unrelated men into the household at all hours), then the investigator must make absolutely clear to the family that the consequences of continuing this situation include the possibility of losing custody of their children. While the looser boundaries may be culturally normative, exposing children to risk is never acceptable.

## Small Size

Sometimes young immigrant children are labeled as "failure to thrive" because of their low weight and small size (Bert Fernández, personal communication, 2002). Children from ethnic groups whose people typically have a smaller stature than people from the dominant culture (including people from the Indian subcontinent, Asians, and Central Americans) may not approach U.S. norms and yet may be perfectly healthy. It would be important to investigate the child's overall health, and not rely on weight and size as sole indicators of growth problems. Additionally, children who breast-feed exclusively typically gain weight in a different pattern than their bottle-fed counterparts (although there are clear advantages to breast-feeding for the babies' health). A breast-feeding child of immigrants may appear "behind" his or her U.S. peers in terms of growth, but this may not be an indication of ill health or neglect (Klass, 2004).

## Appearance and Hygiene

Appearance influences how others see us and how we see them (see Chapter 1 for a discussion of professional dress). From clothing, we may make assumptions about a person's gender, age, occupation, level of hygiene, marital status, sexual orientation, and socioeconomic status. These assumptions can prove problematic if they form part of a child maltreatment assessment and are made without awareness of cultural variations.

Orthodox Jews first cut their children's hair at a party on the child's third birthday. Until this age, a child's hair is allowed to grow freely, so it may look unkempt to the uninformed outsider. Some Muslims, Native Americans, Rastafarians from Jamaica, and members of other ethnic and religious groups have restrictions around the cutting of hair that may make investigators believe the children are poorly groomed when in fact they are groomed in the way their culture dictates. It is important not to penalize families for nonmajority choices in hairstyle. (Of course, dirty hair or lice are another question!)

Additionally, many cultures have restrictions on bathing. During the week after the death of a loved one, Orthodox Jews typically tear their clothing and may not bathe, attend synagogue, work, sit in normal chairs, or look in mirrors. This is intended to help them face their grief, rather than burying it along with the loved one (Orenstein, 1994). Those closest to the person who died are forbidden to cut their hair or shave their beards for a month after the death. Other cultures have similar restrictions related to death, illness, or childbearing. In some cultures, women and girls are told to avoid bathing during menstruation, for fear that it could make them ill.

People from diverse cultures and religions may wear amulets or religious or superstitious objects that puzzle the investigator. A Portuguese man, for instance, may carry a peeled clove of garlic in his pocket at all times to keep away the *mal olhado* (evil eye). Hindu children may wear a thread around their torsos or wrists that should not be removed except in an annual ceremony (Minarik, 1996). Native American children may have markings on their bodies or objects tied onto them, to protect them or to ensure healing after they've been ill (Joe & Malach, 1992). Gypsy (Roma) children and adults usually wear an amulet around their necks (Sutherland, 1996). In infancy, many Latin American and other Roman Catholic children are given necklaces or bracelets with crosses or medallions of saints, which they are instructed never to remove. Investigators should not interpret as problematic what may seem like an unusually strong commitment to the children keeping these objects on their bodies. After all, parents give children these objects to protect them—to show they care. Foster parents should be instructed not to wash off unusual markings, cut off talismans, or remove special necklaces without checking with the parents first. If this is impossible, at the very least these objects should be stored in a safe place.

## Clothing

Many religions require people, sometimes including children, to cover their heads at all times.[1] Some Orthodox Jewish boys wear a yarmulke, or skullcap, on the back of their head. Male Hasidic Jews may wear fur-trimmed or fedora-type hats and heavy coats, even in hot weather, as well as distinctive sidecurls (*payos*). Married Orthodox Jewish women often cover their hair with hats, scarves, or wigs.

Islam requires girls and women to be modest in their dress. Some Muslim women and girls will wear head coverings, ranging from a simple scarf to an elaborate *hijab* that allows only the hands and part of the face to show. Although such practices may be unfamiliar to many investigators, they should not necessarily be regarded as signs of women's oppression within a culture or a family. As Al-Hibri (1999) asks, "Why is it oppressive to wear a head scarf but liberating to wear a miniskirt?" (p. 46). It is important for investigators to refrain from leaping to conclusions about forms of dress that may be unfamiliar to them.

## Responses to Authorities

Immigrant families may respond to child welfare interventions in ways that surprise North American professionals, but the families should not be penalized for their responses. For example:

> A volunteer at a homeless shelter came across a Filipina woman. After speaking with her despite language difficulties, she discovered that the woman's children had been removed from her a year earlier, at which time she became homeless, and she had begun drinking to mute her pain. Her boyfriend had sexually abused one of the children. The police came one day with a child protection worker to remove her children from the home. (With an English-speaking family, most likely the *offender* would have been asked to leave.) The woman was upset to see her children removed by a uniformed policeman and did not understand where they were being taken or why. To protect her

[1]For a more in-depth look at this issue, readers are referred to the wonderful, highly readable text *Culture and Nursing Care: A Pocket Guide* (Lipson, Dibble, & Minarik, 1996), which provides information on specific clothing items used in various cultures (e.g., turbans, veils, and special undergarments).

children, she attacked the police officer and was arrested for assaulting an officer. Her children were removed. Her boyfriend fled and she became homeless and gave up hope of ever seeing her children again. The Union of Pan Asian Communities, a multicultural Asian advocacy organization with professionals from a variety of groups, was able to help her get back up on her feet again, eventually finding housing and helping her get her children back.

That sad story (paraphrased from Okamura, Heras, & Wong-Kerberg, 1995) has a happy ending. Unfortunately, many stories do not.

Many professionals tell families involved with protective services, "The more you cooperate, the better everything is going to turn out." But this advice is not entirely sound; furthermore, it is not necessarily clear what it means "to cooperate." Should families consent to every intervention that is proposed? Should they "voluntarily" give up custody of their children? Clearly, working to achieve the best outcome for one's family requires a combination of acquiescing and asserting one's rights—not an easy task for people who may not speak the language and may not be familiar with the system or the cultural norms at every step.

## Lack of Cooperation

Families are sometimes "punished" by having their children removed because they are seen as unmotivated or uncooperative (Roberts, 2002). Conversely, some children are not afforded adequate protection because abusive parents know how to play the system. Clearly, the more one knows about the workings of the system, the easier it is to follow the (often unwritten) rules, which puts immigrant families and other families who are not from the dominant group at a disadvantage.

There are, of course, many reasons why a family might fail to "cooperate" or comply with a treatment plan, and therefore run the risk of losing custody of their children. For people who do not speak English very well, they may not understand the treatment plan. Even if they understand the words, they may not understand some of the concepts (e.g., "seek developmentally appropriate opportunities"). Chan (1992) describes a Vietnamese mother who attended only intermittently an early intervention program that was deemed essential for the development of her 2½-year-old autistic child. With sensitive inquiry, the professional was able to determine that the mother had not understood what autism was or the importance of the intervention program. (No written information had been provided for her in Vietnamese and the interpreter did not know how to say the word "autism" in Vietnamese.) Additionally, the mother did not feel comfortable intensively stimulating her daughter verbally and socially in the way that was expected in the program—in her culture such stimulation was considered "unnatural and inappropriate" relative to the child's age and level of understanding (p. 227). And finally, the mother was uneasy in the class because of her poor English-speaking skills. Fortunately, she was later given the opportunity to participate in a similar program with other Vietnamese parents, where both she and her child flourished. "Practitioners must avoid using the foster care system as a punishment for [maternal] non-compliance, which reinforces racial oppression" (Woldeguiorguis, 2003, pp. 285–286).

## Unfamiliar Disciplinary Methods

Familiarity with a culture helps us distinguish between punishment techniques that are typical and those that are unusual. If you are not familiar with a given culture's disciplinary norms, I encourage you to seek consultation with professionals who come from the culture in question. Recently, a social worker told me that she had substantiated a charge of child abuse against Mexican American parents who had forced their children to kneel on uncooked rice as a punishment. (This is a common disciplinary practice among some Asian and Latino groups; in Spanish, it is called *hincar*.) Although the mark from the rice on the bare knees vanished quickly and the parents made their children kneel for no longer than 10 minutes at a time, the social worker said the practice seemed so bizarre that she thought it might have been a sign of the parents' mental illness and so she substantiated. A quick call to anyone familiar with Latino cultures or a consultation with a relevant text would have revealed that this disciplinary practice is ubiquitous in many Latin American countries, and should not be considered abusive unless it is used for long periods of time or in unusual ways. (See Chapter 5 for a more developed discussion of this topic.)

## Unfamiliar Medical Interventions

Many traditional medical practices can be mistaken for abuse, including coining, cupping, and moxibustion (see Chapter 2). State protective agencies vary in how they handle these cases. Duong (2003) reports that in California traditional medicine that leaves a mark, such as coining, is not considered a form of child abuse. However, she reports that when a child is found to have bruising caused by a caretaker, even if this is thought to stem from a traditional medical practice, an investigation must be undertaken every time. She explains this policy to parents; she says that by the second or third visit by protective social workers, most Vietnamese, Laotian, and Cambodian parents will forego coining their children to avoid the hassle and suspicion engendered by the visit.

Families from minority cultures may not understand mainstream U.S. medical explanations and practices. Or—in their efforts to provide the care they trust most for their children—they may forego recommended

Western procedures and rely instead on techniques and healers from their own culture. It is not uncommon for Asian families to readjust the dosages of prescription medicine or to stop taking medicine when the symptoms of an illness have disappeared (Chan, 1992), for instance. This fits their traditional view of how illnesses work—as being due to an imbalance of yin and yang. Antibiotics are seen as yang, and so Chinese patients frequently stop taking them when the symptoms vanish. Thus many Chinese parents believe that giving their child antibiotics for too long could make the child overly yang and provoke further problems. If the child's welfare depends on complying with a medical practice, then professionals may well have to enforce its use. But the questioning or rejection of medical care due to cultural beliefs should not be mistaken for simple neglect (see Chapter 2).

## Unfamiliar Practices

Parents may engage in practices with their children that investigators have trouble understanding, and therefore substantiate as abuse. For example:

> I have a friend, Sajjan, who is a practicing Sikh. (Sikhism is a religion from India that believes in one God and the equality of all people.) Sajjan and her family wear white clothes and turbans, they do not cut their hair, they pray several times a day, they keep a vegetarian diet, and they swaddle their children up to age 2 during naptime. "Swaddling" means wrapping a child snuggly in a long blanket or cloth so the child cannot move his or her limbs. In many hospital nurseries in North America new mothers are taught how to swaddle their infants, which comforts the children and helps them sleep. In some ancient societies and today in some parts of the world, infants and toddlers are swaddled too tightly and for such long periods of time that they are deprived of opportunities to explore their environment. Clearly, this overuse of swaddling may be harmful. Sajjan swaddled her children only at naptime. When sleepy, the children would approach her with a swaddling cloth, and gleefully lie down while she rolled them over, wrapped them up, and placed them on their beds. When they awoke they would call out and she would unwrap them. A neighbor saw one of her swaddled toddlers and called protective services. A claim of child abuse was substantiated against her. The investigator later admitted that she was completely unfamiliar with the practice of swaddling and found the house "odd," with its shoes lined up at the door, its people all dressed in white, and the faint scent of incense in the air. She said she substantiated the swaddling as abuse because she had never encountered it before, and her supervisor could not offer her any advice about what to do. Sajjan appealed the ruling. I attended

the hearing on her behalf. Those of us who spoke for Sajjan discussed how happy and well cared for her children were, and how there was no literature claiming any harm from the occasional use of swaddling. I was incredulous when the protective services physician claimed that the swaddling could be considered an abusive form of restraint. In this case, I believe, an unfamiliar but harmless practice was considered child abuse, without regard for its use or its cultural origins, or the health and happiness of all Sajjan's children. Sajjan regretfully agreed to stop swaddling her children and the case was soon closed. She grows tearful, however, when she notes that she is officially considered a "child abuser" in her state.

In another example, in some African cultures children receive ceremonial marking (cuts) on their faces (Qureshi, 1989). A child who has recently returned from a long holiday visiting relatives in Africa may return with these marks. Similarly, some children whose parents follow the Afro-Caribbean religion of *santería* or similar Brazilian practices may be marked with small crosses on their faces or shoulders when they are initiated into the religion. Most jurisdictions would investigate these marks but would not consider them evidence of child abuse (Martínez, 2003) because of the religious context in which they are inflicted.

Adolescent and adult male Shia Muslims from Iran, Iraq, Syria, Lebanon, and other countries may present with multiple bruises or scars, new and old, on the chest or back caused by self-beating with slaps, chains, or small sharp objects such as small knives. These result from a religious ritual to mourn the martyrdom of the grandsons of the prophet Mohammad during the first 10 days of the new Islamic year (Qureshi, 1989). This might be compared to the bruising a Catholic would endure if he or she engaged in self-flagellation or made a pilgrimage to a shrine on his or her knees around the time of Easter. If these bruises were self-inflicted in the context of a religious ceremony, it would be hard to consider them child abuse, unless the child was young, there was substantial coercion involved, or the bruises were such that they left permanent damage.

Recently I took a taxi in New York City that was driven by a loquacious woman from the Dominican Republic. When I told her about my field of interest, she whistled and said, "Oh! If they saw the way I bite my son!" She explained that it is common in her country for a mother to bite her child affectionately, even leaving a mark. She explained this as an expression of the depth of her feeling for her son: "He's so good and I love him so much I could just eat him up!" She said that sometimes her son also bites her back with a similar feeling—it is a game they play, sometimes seeing who can tolerate more pain before pulling his or her arm away. I have seen this practice many times in Latino and Portuguese families. Is it abuse? I'd be hard-pressed to substantiate such a practice as abusive in a family, absent other indicators of problems. However, I advised this mother to consider stopping this biting or doing it more gently, since any teacher or medical professional who noticed teeth marks on her son's arm might feel obligated to report it, and throw her life into more chaos than she can imagine.

## Care of Newborns

Many cultures have strict rules to protect children in the days and weeks immediately after their birth. Infants are often seen as especially vulnerable during this period, requiring special talismans, protection, and prayers so they will not run the risk of being called back into the spirit world. Given the high rates of neonatal mortality which still exist in much of the world, such precautions are understandable. In some cultures, children are not named until they have reached a certain age when they are considered "safe."

Cultures as diverse as the Chinese, the Sikh, and the Somali Bantus will typically require that a mother stay at home with her infant for 40 days after the birth, believing that taking such a young child outside would expose the child to unnecessary risks. Somalis believe that the smells of the world have the potential to make babies sick, so they burn incense twice daily to protect children from these smells. These efforts to shelter newborns from the world can come into conflict with the Western medical system, which often asks mothers to bring in their infants for a 2-week checkup. When possible, an alternative means of meeting this medical requirement should be found, such as arranging for a visiting nurse to attend the mother and infant in their home. Vietnamese mothers will not take a full shower or bath for a month after the birth of a child (Duong, 2003), preferring to clean themselves with a washcloth instead.

Western medicine currently recommends that the umbilical stump be left uncovered and allowed to dry in the days immediately following birth. In many cultures, women are taught to cover or tie the newborn's umbilical stump with materials such as clean cloths, strings, blades of grass, bark fibers, reeds, coins, or roots. These materials can be dangerous if they are unclean or harbor tetanus spores. In most cultures, women are taught to rub the newborn's stump with substances ranging from kohl to animal dung, ash, oil, butter, spice pastes, herbs, and mud. Reasons commonly given for applying a substance to the cord are to keep bad spirits away, to prevent bleeding from the stump, and to promote its drying and separation from the baby (World Health Organization, 1998). Parents' concerns about their newborns' well-being should be honored, but at the same time parents should be taught about standards of hygiene that will protect their babies' health.

## Lack of Information about a Child

Sometimes professionals are surprised that a family may not remember a child's birthday or developmental milestones, and then interpret this as a lack of interest in the child. It is important to remember that what is considered a "milestone" in the dominant Canadian and U.S. cultures may not be considered a "milestone" in the family's culture. For example, Joe and Malach (1992) report that some Native American cultures may be delighted and throw a party when a child first laughs, but not pay attention to the moment when he first learns to sit up or walk. Additionally, they write that talking is considered important somewhere between the child's third and fourth birthday in some Native American cultures, and parents may not notice or pay attention to a child who fails to talk earlier. Traditionally, Somali Bantus do not record or celebrate their children's birthdays, which should not be interpreted as a lack of concern or love for their children.

We must also remember that in many immigrant and low-income families, children may be separated for long periods of time from their parents and raised by other relatives or friends of the family (see Chapter 2). In these cases, parents may not seem to be familiar with their children's histories. Again, this lack of information or contact should not be mistaken for a lack of caring.

## Linguistic Misunderstandings

A tragic case of linguistic misunderstanding in a child abuse assessment was recounted to me by Kee McFarlane (personal communication, May 2003):

> In California, a widower from Laos was raising several small children by himself. The youngest, a preschooler, was exposed to a sexual abuse prevention program at school and disclosed to her teacher that her father slept with her. The child's English was not strong and she may have misunderstood the concepts or been misunderstood by the teacher. Child protective services dispatched an investigator to the home without an interpreter. The father spoke limited English, and— based on what he could understand about the line of questioning— decided that the investigator was looking into possible neglect. The father answered all the questions affirmatively: "Do you sleep with your daughter?" "Yes!" "Do you touch all your children's private parts?" "Yes," the father replied and nodded his head vigorously. He signed a paper listing the claims against him. At a subsequent court hearing, child protective services fought for legal custody of his chil-

dren. When an interpreter explained the charges to the father he was distraught and denied everything, explaining that he had not comprehended the initial investigation. When the judge understood what had happened, he allowed the children to return to the home and informed the father that he would have to attend one more hearing so the charges could be formally dismissed. The father returned home and killed all his children and himself, so deep was his isolation, shame, and confusion over the charges against him.

That is certainly an extreme example. But even in less extreme cases linguistic misunderstandings can lead to tragic outcomes, where parents sign papers they do not understand, where professionals think they understand what a caretaker is saying but do not, and so on (see Chapters 2 and 7 for further discussion of language issues). Investigators should assume they are *not* going to obtain an accurate picture of risk in a family if they cannot speak with the family in its native language. At the very least, a trained professional interpreter should be brought in to help with the assessment.

## One Father, Two Families

In many cultures a man (and particularly a wealthy man) may have more than one family. When François Mitterand, the former prime minister of France, died, both his wife and his mistress of many years attended the funeral, together with their respective offspring. In Latin America, the "official" household may be called the *casa grande* and the unofficial household the *casa chica* (Falicov, 1998, p. 165). While such an arrangement is not exactly socially accepted, it is not condemned with the same vehemence as such an arrangement might be in the United States (where people frequently have extramarital affairs of shorter duration). As long as both households are well cared for economically, and the man is fairly discreet about his second family, all who know about this situation may wink and shrug their shoulders in much of Latin America and some countries in Europe.

In a child abuse investigation, this situation may present when an investigator meets with a woman who describes her "husband," the children's father, and yet is vague about why he is not "home." She may promise that he'll show up for meetings and yet he never does. One possibility, among many, is that he is her common-law husband who also has and lives with another family. Investigators would need to explore this situation with some sensitivity; the children might not know about the father's other family.

In some Muslim cultures, including the Nation of Islam, men may take on more than one wife. While this is relatively rare, investigators may come across Muslim men with multiple wives and their children, often living in the same household. The Quran restricts the circumstances in which polygamy can be practiced, but these edicts are interpreted differently in diverse Muslim communities.

In some religious subgroups, such as some renegade groups of Mormons, a man may also have more than one wife and multiple sets of children, either all living together in the same house or clustered in separate houses in a compound. Investigators would be wise to seek council from their supervisors and the district attorney as to whether these situations are considered a priori problematic for children. The forced marriage of minors (including rape) may also be found in some polygamous sects.

## False Negatives and the Use of Culture as a Justification

Sometimes, professionals can *fail* to recognize a given practice as maltreatment because of cultural differences between the investigator and the family. The professional who holds an excessively relativist position may be inclined to accept as harmless all practices that have a cultural heritage or that a family claims have a cultural heritage. When we look at the many ways people raise children around the globe, we give up our ethnocentric lenses and discover that there is no "one best way" to raise children (Rogoff, 2003). Indeed, cultures successfully meet children's basic needs such as food, shelter, education, and socialization into adulthood in myriad ways. However, this does *not* mean that anything goes, as long as it is "cultural." Some cultural practices are harmful.

For example, in the United States children watch an average of 25 hours of television each week—television that is full of commercials and portrayals of violent acts (Gentile & Walsh, 2002). It could be argued that watching enormous quantities of television is a cultural norm in the United States, and yet few would say this is desirable for children. The same could be said for the U.S. cultural practice of feeding large quantities of fatty foods to children, so that more than 20% of children are obese. Other cultures and nations also engage in cultural practices that are harmful to children, many of which are mentioned in other places in this book. The list includes but is not limited to genital cutting; cures involving contact with mercury, lead, or other toxic substances; punishments that involve ingesting pepper or washing children's mouths out with soap or other irritating substances; corporal punishment; applying animal feces or lead-based kohl to an unhealed umbilical cord; discrimination against girls that results in underfeeding of girl children; child labor, child marriage, child sexual slavery, and prostitution; and so on. Some of these practices are obviously harmful, while others are less obviously harmful. Understanding what is cultural is no easy task. In efforts to be culturally sensitive some instances of harm to a child may be defined as cultural while in fact other risk factors may be present (Maiter, Alaggia, & Trocmé, 2004). Examples of the way this might work are given below.

## Culture as Mask or Smokescreen

A person who knowingly engages in a practice that is harmful to a child will sometimes use a justification that essentially boils down to "my culture made me do it." For example, I worked with a Puerto Rican woman who counted her daughters' pubic hair, had given them douches since they were infants, and inspected their underarms as she tested out various deodorants. She claimed these practices were common in Puerto Rico, where parents were "affectionate" unlike U.S. parents who were cold and distant (Fontes, 1993a). In fact, this behavior would be considered as bizarre and invasive in Puerto Rico as it is on the mainland.

Another example:

> A social worker was investigating physical abuse with a family from the Sicily region of Italy. The father had beaten his daughter, leaving bruises across her face, because she was out past curfew and, in general, he felt unable to control her. The father defended his behavior, claiming that in Sicily no girl would dare defy her parents as his daughter had done, and that he was teaching her a lesson in a way that was appropriate in their culture. The social worker, who was quite knowledgeable about cross-cultural work, was not satisfied with this explanation. Instead, she asked the father what his mother would think about his bruising her granddaughter's face in that way. The father began weeping and admitted that while demanding obedience was culturally acceptable, beating one's daughter in this way would be considered a disgrace. (Sarah Maiter, personal communication, June 2002)

In any case, when hearing a justification of a behavior based on culture, it is important to pay attention to who is defining what qualifies as "cultural." As Okin (1999) points out, cultures are not homogeneous, and the person who is defining what is "cultural" may be the one who is benefiting from the behavior. Frequently, questionable behaviors that are explained away as cultural are behaviors that oppress or restrict women and children (e.g., the veil, genital cutting, wife beating, corporal punishment). So yes, while it may be true that beating one's children is somewhat more common in Portugal than in the United States, a Portuguese family will nevertheless be required to conform to the law where it resides; and certainly not all families in Portugal beat their children. The family's ethnic or national origin may be *part* of the story, but it is not the whole story.

## "My Culture Made Me Do It" and Sexual Abuse

People who sexually offend are apt to use any and all excuses to justify their behavior, and cultural difference is no exception. Some examples:

- "Someone put a curse [or a hex or an evil eye] on me and I didn't know what I was doing. I was not myself. I was in a trance."
- "In my culture all men break in their daughters. I was teaching her how to please her husband."
- "I was showing my son how to be a man; that's what we do in my country."
- "Back home, it is not unusual for young girls to marry older men. That's why I let my best friend have my daughter."
- "We are very hot-blooded. You put a young girl like my stepdaughter in front of us, dressed the way she was dressed, and we can't control ourselves."

Professionals who are accustomed to working with sex offenders will probably be able to sniff out the most egregious of these justifications. When in doubt, the professional should check with another person from the culture in question (while respecting confidentiality).

## ONCE AGAIN: HOW CULTURE MATTERS

Sometimes it doesn't matter whether a given practice is culturally acceptable in terms of determining whether abuse has occurred. In the context of Canadian and U.S. law, families may have to abandon certain practices that were tolerated in their countries of origin. When a practice is culturally acceptable in a country of origin but unacceptable in the United States or Canada, children still need to be protected. However, the notion that the practice was acceptable in the country of origin should be taken into account in assessing the family's overall stability and the most appropriate intervention. For example, let's say a Korean family that recently emigrated uses physically abusive corporal punishment with their children, which is common in Korea (Hahm & Guterman, 2001). Maybe they strike the back of their children's legs with a stick, leaving a mark. It would be entirely appropriate for the parents to have charges of physical abuse substantiated against them. However, if the parents seem amenable to change and did not seem to be aware of the different standards for child raising in their new country, if they do not have other risk factors such as substance abuse or domestic violence, they may not need parenting classes, which are likely to cause them to "lose face," but rather just an occasional contact to make sure they are conforming to the newly learned expectations. It would be important to establish a pathway for the children to seek assistance (e.g., from a school counselor) if the physical abuse recurs.

In other words, the national or ethnic roots of the behavior should be considered relevant in assessing a family and deciding which interventions are most appropriate, but are less apt to be important in determining whether abuse has occurred.

## ASSESSMENT INSTRUMENTS AND STRUCTURED DECISION MAKING

There is a push among practitioners and researchers alike to develop assessment checklists and structured decision-making processes to improve accuracy and formalize child maltreatment assessments. One of the strengths of this approach is that it uses separate instruments to assess for the likelihood of future abuse and future neglect, two forms of maltreatment that appear to have distinct risk factors, although there is some overlap. If well developed, this more formal process should have some distinct advantages over the impressionistic methods many investigators currently use to make decisions about the future of children and families:

• Formal processes provide workers with simple and objective tools to help make the best possible decisions in individual cases. These instruments are based on research and seem more effective than even experienced clinical judgment in distinguishing between families at high and low risk for subsequently abusing children. "In many child welfare agencies, low entry level qualifications, inexperienced workers, minimal training, and high turnover practically guarantee that clinical judgments of risk made by individual workers will vary widely in accuracy. Line staff sometimes fail to identify high risk families during abuse/neglect investigations and therefore do not engage them in service intervention" (Children's Research Center, 2003). Additionally, some cases that are high risk are not opened for services, whereas other low-risk families are carried on caseloads for months or even years. Using these tools should make it easier for less experienced workers to make quality decisions, and for assessments to be conducted with greater efficiency and confidence.

• These tools should also help weed out bias, in that those conducting the assessment answer affirmatively or negatively to fairly objective criteria (e.g., "three or more adults present in the home" or "domestic violence present in the home"). This should increase the reliability and validity of the assessment, that is, the likelihood that the same assessment repeated by a different professional or at a different time would yield the same results, and that the assessment is truly measuring what it purports to be measuring (in this case, risk of future harm to a child). These instruments have the potential for reducing the likelihood that a child's risk status will be misjudged because of the parents' ethnicity or the evaluator's biases. These items chosen have been found to predict future violence across ethnic groups.

- The structured decision-making process should help agencies, supervisors, and individual workers prioritize cases and areas of concern within and among cases. Ideally, this will help focus resources on those clients who need them most. This process should allow for more uniformity in the ways cases are handled across workers, agencies, and municipalities.

The Children's Research Center (2003) of the National Center on Crime and Delinquency identifies the following components of structured decision making:

- *Response priority*, which helps determine if and when to investigate a referral.
- *Safety assessment*, for identifying immediate threatened harm to a child.
- *Risk assessment*, based on research, which estimates the risk of future abuse or neglect.
- *Family needs and strengths assessment*, for identifying problems and establishing a service plan.
- *Case planning and management*, which directly respond to the risk and needs assessments.
- *Case reassessment*, to ensure that ongoing treatment is appropriate
- *Workload-based resource allocation*, assisting agencies to target service resources more efficiently.
- *The role of management information systems*, to support regular monitoring, planning, research, and evaluation.

I share the optimism of the proponents of actuarial risk assessments and structured decision making that these methods may help reduce some of the current ethnic and racial imbalances in the child welfare system (e.g., disproportionate numbers of Black children in out-of-home placements). In a fascinating review of the results of the large-scale implementation of these approaches in California, Georgia, and Michigan, Baird, Ereth, and Wagner (1999) assert that research-based risk assessment contributes to equity in child protective services decision making, in part by reducing some of the "unfettered discretion" (p. 22) that currently characterizes such assessments. This review demonstrates that jurisdictions using actuarial risk assessments do *not* assign more African Americans to high-risk categories, and that the assignment of risk *does* correlate with the likelihood of further maltreatment for both White and Black families (only these two groups were studied).

## CONCLUDING THOUGHTS

The unfairness of current child maltreatment assessment is evidenced by the increasing proportion of Black children who are in the child welfare system and permanently removed from their homes, despite similar rates of abuse across racial groups. The power of the impression will never fully be weeded out of child maltreatment assessments. My hope is that attention to cultural issues, and the implementation of actuarial risk assessments, as discussed here, will assure that child welfare decision making will be based on fair and accurate assessments without bias and prejudice.

### QUESTIONS TO THINK ABOUT AND DISCUSS

1. Describe three cultural minority practices that may be mistakenly considered abusive.

2. Describe three reasons why abusive practices in cultural minority families may be mistakenly assessed as nonabusive.

3. What should a school professional do who has a strong suspicion of child abuse in a family and believes the abusive incident has cultural roots? Should he or she file a report with child protective services?

4. Describe a couple of the ways your own background influences your assessment of others' practices as abusive or nonabusive. Give specific examples, if possible, from your own professional or personal life.

5. How might structured decision-making processes and formal assessment instruments make decision making about child maltreatment less prone to cultural bias?

# CHAPTER FOUR

# Interviewing Diverse Children and Families about Maltreatment

This chapter discusses interviewing culturally diverse children about possible child maltreatment. While it focuses on the kind of forensic interview that professionals conduct in children's advocacy centers and police stations, the information is relevant to social workers, medical staff, attorneys, guardians ad litem, psychologists, and professionals who work in other settings.

Speaking with children and families about possible maltreatment is difficult and stressful. The interviewer tries to help children focus their conversation without leading them. Other professionals may be watching from behind a one-way mirror, and the interview may be audio- or videotaped for use in court. The interviewer is often under pressure to complete the process quickly and obtain all the necessary information in just one session. Interviewers know their work may directly influence criminal prosecutions, family integrity, and children's safety and mental health. If the child discloses abusive incidents, the material is often painful for the interviewer as well as for the child. As a disclosure of abuse unfolds, many interviewers find themselves experiencing a heavy feeling in the pit of their stomach and holding the vague notion that it would be so much easier just to "not go there." Indeed, many professionals *avoid* speaking about child abuse with adults and children or cut short the conversation before the client is ready.

To complicate matters further, the child may have a limited language ability, may have been threatened into keeping secrets, may be suffering from trauma, and may be frightened and intimidated by the entire process. Children do not know the interviewers and often wonder why they should trust them with their scariest secrets. When language and cultural differences enter into the mix, achieving enough rapport to elicit full and accurate information may seem to be nearly impossible.

However, interviewers don't simply throw up their hands in despair, because they care about children, and because they know that obtaining the information is necessary to protect this child and other children from future abuse. Successful interviewers adjust the process according to the child's culture, background, and living context. This chapter details ways to make these adjustments.

Successful interviewers also adjust their approaches according to the child's age and developmental level. Preschoolers may warm up quickly to an interviewer who speaks in a singsong voice, carries a basketful of crayons, and is all smiles. Teenagers, on the other hand, are apt to turn their back on interviewers who approach them with even a hint of condescension. As children advance developmentally, their relationship to their parents' culture and to the dominant culture may also change. The intersections of individual development and culture is integrated in the discussion below.

Because of the lack of literature in this area, the suggestions I am making have not been supported by empirical research. Although there is extensive recent research on interviewing, most of it ignores cultural issues. Therefore these suggestions are based on my own clinical experience, my research on cultural issues in sexual child abuse, my reading of multicultural literatures in various fields, and reported experiences of the many dozens of forensic interviewers whom I've trained and with whom I've spoken over the years.

## BEFORE THE INTERVIEW OR FIRST SESSION

### Gathering Information

Whenever possible, gather information about the child's cultural background before you meet with him or her. Racial information is not enough, since culture is not defined by skin color. For instance, the culture of a Black person from Jamaica is different from that of an African American person in New York City. A White person whose family has lived for many generations in Texas has a different culture from a White person whose parents have recently emigrated from Russia. If you have the time, do some background reading on the child's cultural group before meeting. (See the References at the back of this book for suggestions.)

It is important to assess how much the child is integrated into the dominant U.S. culture, and how much he or she retains of the culture of origin. Try to gather some of this information from other providers before your first contact with the child. Answers to the following questions may be helpful:

- What language or languages are spoken at home? It is important not to make assumptions about this issue. For instance, some people from Ecuador speak Quechua, some people from Bolivia speak Aymara, and some people from Mexico speak Nahuatl, Maya, or a host of other indigenous languages, rather than Spanish.
- What language does the child prefer to speak with siblings and friends?
- Is the child an immigrant or the child of an immigrant? If so, from where, and what were the circumstances of immigration? (See Chapter 2 for more information.)
- Who lives at home? Who else stays there?
- What do the adults do for a living?
- What is the child's religion and how observant is the child's family in regard to practicing that religion?

Answers to some of the above questions will help you understand the extent to which the child is embedded in his or her ethnic minority culture, and how much of an adjustment you therefore may need to make to your standard interviewing process.

## Location of the Interview

Some professionals have no choice about where they conduct their interviews, while others do. Guidelines recommend that interviews be conducted in a neutral environment. However, they rarely explain what characteristics make an environment neutral, and for whom. What is a "neutral environment" for an African American child whose father is on the police force? What is a neutral environment for a Mexican American preschooler who does not speak English and has never interacted intimately with someone who does not speak Spanish? Schoolage children are frequently interviewed at school, but they may not see their school as a neutral environment, especially if they are discriminated against in school and feel alienated from it.

Given that there may be no truly neutral environment suitable for all children, interviewers must do the best they can. If they have the possibility of interviewing "off-site," interviewers may be able to offer two or three choices to the child, finding out where he or she would rather meet. For example, an interviewer could offer either to meet the child in a private room at school or to bring the child down to his or her office. People who frequently conduct interviews in the field are encouraged to develop a variety of interview sites in places that may be familiar to children from different ethnic groups, including places of worship, schools, hospitals, children's advocacy centers, and Head Start centers. Interviewers who work in areas that are racially, culturally, or economically segregated should be sure to establish a number of possible interview locations within each community. Children will be uncomfortable if they have to enter an unknown neighborhood to talk about something scary and threatening.

If police are involved in the interview, they should be dressed in plain clothes and should not carry a gun. The child and his or her family should be protected from seeing scenes that may be frightening and intimidating (e.g., seeing armed officers or people in handcuffs or shackles). Members of many ethnic groups do not see police as friendly allies because they have had difficult encounters with law enforcement and the military in this and other countries. In situations where children have to be transported large distances for their interviews, as often occurs with children living on American Indian reservations, a trustworthy person who is familiar to the child should accompany him or her to the interview.

If you have control over the space where you conduct your work, try to make it child-friendly and inviting to people from different cultures (see Chapter 9). Many immigrant children live sheltered lives at home with their families and may be accustomed to a small neighborhood and a set routine. Interviewers should take extra time to orient the child to the place where the interview is held, and ask the child how he or she feels in the room. Allow a young child to bring a toy, a blanket, or some other comfort object to the interview.

Interviewers should explain the use of video cameras, mirrors, microphones, and any other equipment that may be unfamiliar to the child. Children who come from families with little or no high-tech equipment might be less comfortable with the process. Some interviewers avoid telling children that their interviews are being recorded or observed because of their concern that such information would intimidate the child and make him or her less likely to disclose. I feel strongly that we have a moral and ethical obligation to tell children about the process in which we are asking them to participate (in a way that is developmentally appropriate). First, they have the right to refuse to participate. And second, if they have been abused, they have had acts done to them without their full knowledge and informed consent. We must avoid repeating this kind of betrayal, even if we mean well. Finally, if children later discover that their words or images were recorded without their knowledge, they will feel misled and will be less likely to cooperate with an investigation or intervention.

Interviewers who take notes during their conversations should explain what they are writing and why. They can say, "What you are telling me today is really important. I am writing it down so I won't forget any of it." Especially for children whose parents are not very literate, the act of taking notes may seem strange and off-putting.

## Ethnic Matching

Ethnic minority children are bicultural to varying degrees. Most children are exposed to people from the dominant culture on television, but for some this is virtually their only contact. Others may live in a neighborhood populated largely by people from the dominant culture, and may have no contact with other people from their own ethnic minority group. The less comfortable a child is with the dominant culture, the more important it may be for the child to be interviewed by someone from the same cultural group.

Some preliminary but highly provocative research suggests that it is particularly difficult for Black children to disclose a "negative secret" about a Black person to a White interviewer (Dunkerley & Dalenberg, 1999). This was not simply a question of same versus different—White children did not show effects to nearly the same degree in terms of disclosing a secret to a Black versus a White interviewer. While this research is far from conclusive, it does underscore the importance of diversity in interviewers so that ethnic matching can be implemented where indicated.

Sometimes a child will be hostile and silent with a specific professional either because of past negative experiences, because of prejudice, or because the professional reminds the child of the abuser. In these cases, if the interviewer cannot obtain information or establish a productive working relationship, it may be helpful to suggest that the child meet with another professional, perhaps one who differs from the original interviewer in demographic characteristics (e.g., gender, race, age).

## Accompanying Adults

Sometimes families will want to bring a spiritual leader, a godparent, or a more acculturated relative to official situations such as child abuse interviews. They can often accompany the family to the meeting and offer them support in the waiting room. However, interviewers need to use their judgment about meeting with individuals without the escort. I have heard stories about professionals who unwittingly interviewed a battered woman about child abuse in the presence of her battering husband or his close relative. Sometimes the batterer even serves as interpreter. Obviously, the information obtained under such circumstances is suspect.

What is the role of parents or other adults who might accompany a child to an interview? On the one hand, a parent who thoroughly supports a child's disclosure and gives the child the go-ahead to respond to questions is priceless. On the other hand, children may skip critical details to spare their parents distress. For instance, I worked with a girl who had disclosed a brutal vaginal rape to a detective while knowing that her mother was behind the mirror. However, she did *not* disclose that she was also raped anally because she thought this would disgust her mother. Months later, the day before she was due to testify in court, she finally revealed the anal rape to me, her psychotherapist. The new information required a new set of charges and delayed the case for months, which created additional stress for everyone, especially the child. If her mother had not been behind the mirror for the initial interview, perhaps the girl would have disclosed this part of her assault earlier. Children should not be interviewed with a family member in the room or behind the mirror (APSAC, 2002).

An immigrant parent, and particularly the parent of a child who has been abused, may not want to let the child out of his or her sight, even for an interview. The interviewer should explain carefully the reasons he or she wishes to meet with the child alone, and try to be respectful of the parent's concerns. The interviewer should explain exactly what will happen during the interview. If there is to be a physical exam, the interviewer should explain why, exactly what will be done, and who will do it. If a girl needs a genital exam, many parents prefer that it be performed by a female medical professional. Whenever possible, this wish should be respected. Parents are frequently concerned that girls might "lose their virginity" (i.e., have their hymen torn) in the process of an examination. Very concrete information may be helpful. For example, show the parents the instruments (e.g., a colposcope), say that they will not penetrate the child, explain that the exam will not hurt, and so on. The person who orients the child to the exam should explain that no "shots" will be given, and that most children do fine with the exam—it doesn't bother them at all.

Although parents usually cannot be in the room with children during interviews, children—and particularly immigrant children—are still more likely to speak openly if their nonoffending parents explicitly tell them to do so. In many Latino and Asian American families, children are taught to sacrifice themselves for the good of the family. If they believe disclosing is a selfish act that will destroy the family, they will not speak. Interviewers would do well to find a nonoffending family member or member of the community—for example, a mother, grandmother, or aunt—who can encourage the child to speak openly and honestly. Even when these family members do not believe that abusive acts have occurred, they often can be persuaded to ask a child to tell the truth.

The nonoffending parent should be told about the importance of his or her support for the child's truth telling. In some cases, of course, this will not be possible. Sometimes another family or community member such as a cousin, teacher, doctor, nurse, psychotherapist, social worker, or victim witness advocate can encourage the child to speak openly. Of course, confidentiality needs to be observed.

For an interviewer to build rapport with any child, but particularly with a child who differs from the interviewer culturally, the interviewer needs to establish at least a cordial relationship with the adult who accompanies the child. The interviewer should take some time to orient the adult to the process and demonstrate to the child that the adult is comfortable with him or her. People from many cultures need some chitchat time to get familiar with professionals. The professional can discuss the weather or ask about their trip to the interview site. Interviewers should not view this orientation as a waste of time. Trying to get right down to business may result in more frustration over the long term.

If an accompanying adult needs to wait while a child is interviewed, the adult should be allowed to sit in a private or neutral place that is not clearly identified as being associated with child maltreatment, so that he or she will not be seen by neighbors and can avoid losing face. People who live in small, tight-knit ethnic communities may be especially concerned about being seen in settings that will create gossip.

Enlisting a child's cooperation in an interview is by no means a straightforward process, particularly where there are cultural differences between the interviewer and the child. It may seem self-evident to the interviewer that the child should reveal sensitive information and that this revelation will lead to helpful interventions. This is by no means self-evident to children (or adults) from many communities.

In some cultures personal matters are discussed indirectly, if at all. The more that is left unsaid, the better. In fact, in Spanish there is a saying, "*La mejor palabra es la que no se dice*" (The best word is the one that is left unsaid). Similarly, Ide (1995) writes, "In Japanese communication, people expect others to guess about a certain unstated part of the message. . . . In effect, it is a receiver's responsibility to be sensitive to the speaker's true message" (p. 26). In Japanese, the term *ishin denshin* describes the idea of an immediate and direct communication between two minds which does not need words (Morsbach, 1988). From a Japanese perspective, an interviewer who insists on direct explicit statements may be showing a striking lack of skill as a listener. If explicit statements are needed for a legal case, the interviewer may need to request this overtly.

Keeping sensitive and shameful matters quiet may be seen as a virtue, permitting everyone involved to avoid public shaming and to save face. To gain a child's cooperation, the professionals may need to persuade the child and the accompanying adult(s) of the good that will be accomplished by revealing the truth. This persuasion will be suspect if it is too strong-handed. It will take gentle calm and time to win this trust.

Children from many cultural groups are raised not to speak to an adult unless spoken to. In Puerto Rico and Cuba there is an expression, "*Los niños hablan cuando las gallinas mean,*" which means that children are to speak when hens pee. Apparently, hens do not urinate, and by implication children should not speak. Many cultures have a version of this expression (e.g., "Children should be seen and not heard"). If children do not respond readily to interviewers' requests for information, this may be due to cultural proscriptions rather than to fear or instructions to hide information.

Depending on their country of origin, immigrant children—even teenagers—may be unwilling to discuss information with an interviewer without a parent's express permission (Lipson, 1993). Often children raised in households with strict discipline will turn to a parent or another familiar adult to see if they are permitted to speak. For instance, an interviewer might ask the child a simple question, such as his age, and the child might look at his mother and answer only after she nods. Or the adult might consistently answer questions that are directed at the child. This is not necessarily an indication that they are concealing a secret or lying. Rather, the children are unaccustomed to having adults turn to them for information and—out of respect—allow their parents to control the conversation.

## BUILDING RAPPORT AND ESTABLISHING TRUST

### Empathy and Warmth

Mainstream North American professionals are often seen as cold and distant. I suggest that interviewers make a special effort to demonstrate warmth and show that they care. In Spanish, the applicable term is *personalismo*. A professional demonstrates *personalismo* by showing clients a *personal and specific* caring for them. One Puerto Rican woman whom I interviewed, who had been in therapy for sexual abuse, offered the following advice:

> "The most important thing is spiritual and moral support. Let the person know that you really care for him or her. We Latinos, we are affectionate. We like that kind of attention and love, understanding, and trust, so you won't be afraid to speak. It's hard for us to say for the first time, 'I need help.'"

Some interviewers are concerned about how much of a positive connection they should establish with a child during an investigative interview. They may worry that too much of a link could be construed as leading the child. Interestingly, however, research by Davis and Bottoms (2002) shows that the *warmer* the connection established between the interviewer and the child, the more comfortable the child will be in correcting the interviewer when the interviewer makes a mistake. Also, the child tends to supply more information and more correct information. There is no danger in establishing a warm relationship with the child per se—the danger lies in rewarding specific responses.

An interviewer who deliberately withholds warmth and connectedness is not apt to get far with a child, especially with a child who may come from an affectionate culture. While threats and intimidation may push an adult criminal suspect to reveal information, they are not appropriate or effective with children.

I once conducted a forensic interview training that was attended by several Puerto Rican professionals from the island. They were surprised to witness the hands-off, monotone manner of the U.S. interviewers. They said that a Puerto Rican child would interpret this manner as cold, disinterested, and rejecting. The child would suspect that the interviewer disliked him or her, and therefore would be reluctant to answer questions. Some of the most skilled interviewers I have seen are former elementary schoolteachers who exude warmth and know how to help children relax. Conveying warmth and friendliness may be particularly important for children from cultures where adults routinely interact personably with them.

## Establishing Your Identity

Depending on their culture, the family may trust some providers but not others. Many Asian fathers will have more trouble trusting a young female social worker than they would an older male doctor. Many women, however, may be more comfortable discussing sexual matters with a woman than with a man. Additionally, many immigrants and members of conservative religious groups simply refuse to allow their daughters to be alone in a room with a male professional. Where possible, this desire should be respected and a woman provider should be called in.

To gain trust, professionals should explain their roles carefully, as well as their credentials and their experience. If the interviewer is not from a group that the client trusts easily, it may take some time to build rapport. Professionals should try not to rush the process.

Be clear with adults and children about the purpose of the conversation. Are you looking for facts for a court case, or are you intending to help the child avoid long-term trauma? Explain the purpose in plain terms—to someone who is not in the field, the terms "investigation," "assessment," "evaluation," "examination," and "interrogation" may all sound the same.

Many immigrants and low-income people have trouble distinguishing among various agencies and professional roles. The system may seem like a large, intimidating structure, designed to investigate them, do them harm, destroy their families, and keep them down. Many people—including children—will worry about where the information they give you could end up and how it could be used. Could it:

- Get them or someone in their family deported?
- Cause food stamps, welfare, or unemployment benefits to be cut off, or cause them to lose their housing?
- Cause them or someone they love (or fear) to end up in jail?
- Destroy their family?

Interviewers should explain their role carefully, and allow the child and accompanying adult to ask questions. Interviewers should be honest in their responses. Unfortunately, interviewers cannot always guarantee that everything will be okay. Interviewers should only make promises that they can keep.

## DURING THE INTERVIEW

### Acknowledging Taboos

Interviewers should keep in mind the strong cultural and religious rules against "talking dirty." In Latin cultures, talking about sex is generally considered *muy bajo*, a low thing to do. One Latina woman I interviewed for a study said that her family's attitude was like this: "If it occurs to you to say your uncle touched you, or even to think [about saying] it, watch out! Where are you going to go if not to heaven?" Speaking about sexual acts, even in the context of an interview, may seem almost as dirty as engaging in them.

A Puerto Rican woman I interviewed who had been abused for years as a child said she would have disclosed to any adult who seemed comfortable talking about sex, but no one did. It is extremely difficult for most people to discuss sexual matters—even with the people they love, with whom they may have shared a bed for years. And yet we expect children to discuss sexual acts with someone they don't know who has power over them. With this in mind, the following strategies may help:

• Interviewers should increase their own comfort in speaking about sex and other sensitive topics by practicing. They should conduct role-play interviews with a colleague in front of a video camera, and then critique each other's work. If they ordinarily video- or audiotape their interviews, they should obtain supervision from their superiors and from their peers on these tapes. If they conduct interviews in front of a one-way mirror, they should ask a trusted colleague to observe a session and take notes exclusively for supervision purposes. The best interviewers receive frequent feedback about their work, and adjust what they do accordingly.

• Interviewers should assure children that it is okay to talk about these matters in this setting. If a child seems to be struggling over how to say something, the interviewer can offer some reassurance such as "Go ahead" or "It's all right." Some children and even some adults have so internalized the rules about not using "garbage-can words" that they feel themselves unable to speak about something that happened "down there." They may describe an unwanted rape as "He made love to me" because they simply do not have other words to describe it, or are reluctant to use them.

• Interviewers should assure children that they are expected to tell the truth, and it will not make the interviewer angry or shocked or embarrassed.

In investigative interviews, it may be important to pursue information persistently, even if it *is* sensitive for cultural reasons. If an interviewer fails to pursue information adequately, the children may be left vulnerable to further abuse. If the interviewer has the impression that a child does not wish to discuss exactly what happened during a sexual encounter, and has the impression that the child has been taught that talking about sex is bad, depending on the child's age the interviewer can ask the child to draw or write about it. Let the child know that the details are important.

## Discussing Difficult Issues

Depending on their role, interviewers may want to elicit detailed information about the alleged abuse and the context surrounding it. However, this goal conflicts with common cultural notions about keeping shameful issues within the family. Interviewers should be alert to signs that the child is uncomfortable discussing sensitive issues. Interviewers can give children a signal to use when they know the answer to something but are uncomfortable talking about it. For example:

> "I'm going to ask you a lot of questions because I need to know things that only you can tell me. And I might ask you something that makes you uncomfortable, that you don't want to talk about now. If you know the answer, please try to answer it. But if you feel like you just don't want to, but you *do* know the answer, I want you to give me a

signal. You can just raise up your little finger like this [the interviewer demonstrates]. Let me see you do that. Good. Now what are you supposed to do if I ask you a question that you know the answer to, but don't want to answer now?"

In this way, if you ask questions that the child is uncomfortable discussing, he or she can let you know. Then you may be able to talk about why the child feels uncomfortable, and try to alleviate his or her concerns around it.

Children may be uncomfortable discussing things for reasons the interviewer might not suspect. For example, a child could be uncomfortable about specifying the race of the alleged assailant because he or she has been told it is bad to talk about someone's race. Or the child might be uncomfortable discussing a situation because it involved alcohol, and for religious reasons he or she believes the parent should not have been drinking. Sometimes children from minority cultures are embarrassed to describe cultural activities—like making tortillas or playing mahjong. And, of course, children are uncomfortable answering questions that they believe imply that they did something wrong. For instance, if they saw pornography or cooperated in sexual activity, they may feel guilty.

I watched a forensic interview in which a 5-year-old Mexican American girl was interviewed in English about her experiences of abuse by her stepfather. She provided a great deal of information and did not hesitate until the interviewer asked if the stepfather *said* anything while he did these acts. (The interviewer was trying to establish sexual intent.) The little girl nodded. The interviewer asked what he said. She said, "He said those things you call people when you're mad at them." The interviewer asked what those things were and the little girl looked embarrassed and said, "I mean, he didn't say anything."

Several issues become evident here. First, the girl may not know what those words mean, although she senses that they are "bad" words. Second, she is unlikely to know how to say those words in English. Third, she has undoubtedly been taught never to say those words. The interviewer just moved on. If the interviewer had been more in tune with the language issues, she could have asked what language the stepfather was speaking. If the girl said, "Spanish," she could have asked the girl to say those words in Spanish, adding, "It's okay to use any kind of word here."

## Questioning

Adults ask children questions for different reasons in different cultures. They ask questions to reinforce a lesson, such as "Where are you supposed to be when it gets dark?" They ask questions to show love, such as "Are you cute?" Adults often ask children questions to show what they know.

For example, "What time is it when the big hand is on the 12 and the little hand is on the 3?" Children are often asked questions as a social gesture, as in "Do you know what happened to me today?" And—as may be familiar to readers with teenagers at home—adults often ask questions as a reprimand: "Just what is that wet towel doing on the living-room couch?" These questions serve important social functions, but they are not attempts to gather information. Adults rarely ask children questions for which they do not already know the answer. It may take time for children to get used to the idea that the interviewer is asking questions to gather information.

The interviewer's first purpose is to encourage the child to talk. The interview should not feel like a test or an interrogation. Particularly with younger children and children for whom English is a second language, the first questions should be short, simple, and mostly open-ended. Initial questions that start with "Tell me about . . . ," such as "Tell me about what happened when you got home from school yesterday" or "Tell me what happens when your father gets angry," are especially useful. The interviewer is training children to speak in their own words with as much detail as possible. Although the interview may be a strange situation for a child, storytelling is a common practice for children from all cultures. A well-placed prompt can be helpful, such as "Tell me what happened from the beginning until the end. Don't leave anything out." If open-ended questions are not eliciting information, interviewers will need to move on to appropriate focused questions (Faller, 1999; Reed, 1993).

Interviewers should train children to correct them if they say something wrong in the interview context. Correcting an adult is a taboo for many children, particularly for those from cultures where they are taught not to question adults. Reed (1993) suggests the following kind of statement:

> Sometimes I get mixed up and say the wrong thing. I need your help so I don't say the wrong thing. If I do say the wrong thing, will you please tell me? Just say, "That's not right" or, "You made a mistake," okay? (p. 8)

This kind of statement is more useful if followed by a role play where the child has an opportunity to "catch" the adult making a mistake (e.g., misnaming a cartoon character that the child has already identified correctly).

## Verb Tenses

Depending on their age, many children have trouble with the tenses of verbs. They will tell what happened in the present tense, or they will use nonstandard forms of verbs. This is especially true for children who speak more than one language, including African American Vernacular English. A child might say, "He ask me to touch his weewee so I go do it." Interviewers should not interrupt the child to ask about the timing or to affirm that this happened in the past, yesterday morning. Instead, interviewers should listen to the story and then ask specific questions for clarification if necessary. Children who are continually interrupted are apt to feel judged and may withdraw into themselves, refusing to continue speaking.

Children who are not native speakers of English may have difficulty with complex verb forms like "would have," "should have," "may have," and so on, to say nothing of constructions like: "Where were you when you first told someone that something happened to you in the tent behind your aunt's house?" Interviewers should keep their questions short and direct, using no embedded clauses. Every few minutes, interviewers should ask if the child understands the questions. If the interviewer has the sense that the child does not understand, the interviewer should pause the interview and try to ascertain what is happening. Interviews with young children and children who are nonnative speakers of English can be incredibly slow, requiring a great deal of time and patience on the part of the interviewer.

## Interviewing Aids

For the cultural reasons discussed above, because they are young or are verbally impaired, or because they have been threatened, many children are unwilling or unable to *say* what happened. However, some may be willing to *show* the interviewer nonverbally if supplied with the means to do so. Interviewing aids can help.

## Drawings

When children are having trouble talking, or after they have completed a verbal disclosure, interviewers can ask them to draw what they are describing. The child's drawings may be admissible in court as evidence. Once I worked with a 10-year-old girl whose father had been jailed twice for molesting children outside the family. This young girl had never been assessed properly about whether he had molested her too. I was assigned as the therapist to help the family reintegrate the father as he returned from prison. The parents did all they could to keep me from meeting with their children. With the help of the man's probation officer, I finally met with the older daughter alone.

Almost immediately she said, "I know you're going to try to make me say something bad about my dad, but I won't because he didn't do anything." I tried to build trust with her but also felt an urgent need to protect her and her little sister if anything *was* going on. I finally asked her to draw a picture of her family doing something (a kinetic family drawing [Burns & Kaufman, 1972]). She drew herself and her sister in shorts and tummy shirts with mouths wide open, their arm up and their bellies exposed, with terror in their eyes. She drew her 4-year-old sister with huge breasts. She verbally continued to deny any kind of abuse, but through the pictures I came to believe she was pointing to another possible source of information: her sister. I quickly set up an interview for the little sister with one of my colleagues who was an experienced forensic interviewer, not the family therapist. The little girl walked into the session and declared, "I can't tell you anything because my father will kill me." She ended up disclosing multiple instances of abuse perpetrated against herself and her sister. The older girl's drawing provided information that she was not willing to provide verbally. It should he noted, however, that trying to diagnose abuse purely on the basis of a child's drawings has not been found to be accurate.

A drawing in the child's own hand with his or her own words may be enough to make an offender confess or reach a plea, saving the child the further trauma of the court process. In the video series *Investigative Interviewing Techniques in Child Sexual Abuse Cases* (Chesapeake Institute, 1993), Detective Richard Cage demonstrates how he used a child's drawing to gain the support of the nonoffending mother and the confession of the offending father.

## Anatomical Drawings

Interviewers often ask children to point to body parts on anatomical drawings—outlines of the fronts and backs of human figures. These outlines should be without obvious racial characteristics, such as long hair for women. Some interviewers have a variety of drawings available of people of different ages and ethnic backgrounds. Others prefer to use a vague human outline, like a gingerbread figure. Interviewers can point to body parts and ask children what they call each part (e.g., "hair," "titty"), and what they call it at home, if they speak another language at home. The interviewers should write down these names. Establishing the names during the relatively neutral conversation about the drawing can save mishaps and misunderstandings later during the course of a disclosure. For instance, in English many girls use "bottom" to refer to their vagina and anus, and in Spanish many girls use "*pompis*" for the same two parts. It may be helpful, during a disclosure, to turn back to the drawing and say, "Remember, this is the front and this is the back. You said he touched your bottom. Circle where he touched you. Do you have another name for that?"

## Dolls

Pressure from defense attorneys has caused interviewers to be extremely cautious about using dolls in investigative interviews because children grow up using dolls primarily for imaginative play. However, research has demonstrated that, when used judiciously, dolls can help children describe true events that they might otherwise fail to discuss (APSAC, 1995). Some interviewers choose to use dolls after a disclosure has been established to gather the details about specific incidents, to clarify information, or to allow children distance from their body in their recounting of the incidents (Holmes & Vieth, 2003). Young children can sometimes demonstrate effectively on dolls body positions or details of abusive incidents that are difficult for them to describe in words. Many interviewers find that ordinary dolls or even teddy bears that are not anatomically correct work as well as anatomically correct dolls in many circumstances.

If interviewers are using dolls, they should have them available in a variety of races, sizes, and apparent ages. The interviewers should not make assumptions about which dolls the child will use based on the child's own race or ethnicity. The child should be permitted to select the dolls him- or herself and say who each doll is representing.

The value of dolls—used judiciously—was driven home to me recently when I watched a heartbreaking videotape of a kindergartener who disclosed sexual abuse by her father. She provided all the relevant information quite well. Her English was not completely fluent, however, and she struggled with prepositions (e.g., "on," "in," "over"), as many nonnative speakers do. She was permitted to show the interviewer—using anatomically correct dolls—how her father positioned her and what he did with their clothing when he raped her. After she finished demonstrating quite clearly to the interviewer (and the video camera), she then proceeded to show how her uncle positioned her when *he* raped her. It is certainly possible that the girl would have eventually revealed information about the other person who offended against her in the course of the interview, but the way in which this information was revealed spontaneously by the child with the use of dolls was vivid and convincing. The interviewer immediately put away the dolls and said, "Let's talk about your uncle now." The interviewer proceeded to gather as much information as she could verbally regarding the uncle, before returning to the dolls again. In this case, in their jurisdiction, the district attorney was able to present the videotape in court as evidence, and the two men were convicted. The dolls were invaluable in obtaining a precise picture of the abuse that had occurred.

## Other Media

Interviewers who use other media, such as puppets or dollhouses, should try to make sure they fit the child's circumstances. For instance, a child who lives in a one-bedroom apartment may have trouble using a large, multilevel dollhouse to show where abuse occurred.

## Crime Scene Information and Physical Abuse

In any investigative interview, it can be helpful to identify and locate items that could be used by law enforcement. Corroborating physical evidence may take the burden of the case off the shoulders of the child. This is always important, but particularly so when the child is young, developmentally delayed, or less verbally expressive for some other reason. Most people are familiar with the idea of gathering physical evidence in cases of sexual abuse, and so they inquire about pornographic pictures and stained clothing, for example. However, interviewers frequently neglect to think about physical evidence when handling other kinds of child maltreatment, such as physical abuse.

One study in a single hospital showed that children had been physically abused by more than 100 different instruments (Showers & Bandman, 1986). The use of these instruments varied by culture: African American children were more likely to be struck with a belt, strap, switch, stick, or electric cord, while White American children were more likely to be struck by a board, paddle, or open hand. Often interviewers may neglect to ask about evidence of physical abuse because they are from a different culture than that of the child, and it doesn't occur to them that objects may form part of the abuse (see Chapter 5).

An interviewer who is concerned about physical abuse in the home can ask the child what happens when he or she does something wrong, and what happens when the grownups get angry at home. If the child mentions abusive punishment with specific objects, the interviewer can ask where these are stored. When law enforcement gathers physical evidence, the case does not rest entirely on the child's testimony.

## Language Issues

Interviewers should not confuse language competency with competency to testify or with intelligence. A child may not be competent to testify in English, but may be competent to testify in another language.

There are four options for conducting interviews with children whose native language is not English: conduct the interview in English only, conduct it in the child's first language only, use an interpreter, or have a bilingual interviewer conduct the interview. I will examine each of these options.

## Interviewing in English Only

If the child seems fluent enough in English, the interviewer may be able to proceed in English only. This is certainly the easiest option for interviewers who do not speak the child's first language, but it can cause problems. In workshops, sometimes I ask for a show of hands of people who have studied a language other than English. Usually almost everyone in a room raises their hand. Then I ask them to turn to someone they have never met and tell that person about their most embarrassing or frightening experience in that other language. Giggles usually abound. I point out that this is what we are asking children to do when we ask them to disclose in a language that is not their first language, the language of their heart. We are asking too much of children when we are asking them to reveal sensitive information and overcome linguistic challenges at the same time.

Even children who seem fluent in English are apt to use the words of their first language to discuss intimate matters and body parts. For example, when my son Gabriel was 3, he spoke English best, but also understood Portuguese. When we were alone with him, my husband and I spoke to him in Portuguese, but he spoke English with his sisters and at preschool. If anyone had needed to conduct an investigative interview with him, he or she would probably have failed to consider the possibility that he might need a bilingual interviewer. But the only time he ever heard the word for "penis," as far as we know, was in the bathtub, and then it was always in Portuguese. He would not have been able to respond to a question about his penis in English unless the interviewer either knew the word for it in Portuguese or was sensitive to the fact that he might have an unusual name for it. This is just one simple example of how language issues can be more important than they first appear.

We know little about memory and language. If a child experiences an assault in one language but is interviewed about it in another, we don't know how this affects her ability to access her memories. Often, immigrant teenagers and older children will claim they can speak English well and consent to be interviewed in English. Their English language abilities may be a point of pride. However, their answers in English may be hesitant and halting—a problem that frequently disappears when they are given a chance to speak in their native tongue.

Even if an interviewer chooses to conduct the interview in English, if the child is bilingual, it would be best for the interviewer to be bilingual also. If not, an interpreter should be on hand to fill in occasional words, as the need arises (see Chapter 7).

In one forensic interview, a teenager requested a Spanish-speaking interviewer. None was available so she was interviewed in English with an interpreter present. The girl scoffed at the idea of needing an interpreter since she spoke English in school every day. However, as the interview progressed, the team noticed that she would give one answer to a question in English, and then, when the question was repeated in Spanish, she'd supply a different answer. In other words, her English was not quite as fluent as she thought. In some jurisdictions law enforcement personnel conduct all forensic interviews with teenagers, and they often assume that teenagers will be able to handle themselves in English. I urge caution in making this assessment based on a teenager's apparent bravado. Language obstacles frequently emerge for nonnative speakers who speak English, especially in tense situations where precision is important. Even children who are highly bilingual may tire as an interview progresses, and lose some of their fluency in English if it is their second language.

## Interviewing in the Child's First Language Only

Children can be interviewed in their first language (other than English) only, if the person conducting the interview speaks the child's first language fluently or almost fluently. For instance, an officer who speaks Korean could interview a child in Korean. However, it is important that people with limited English proficiency receive the same quality interview as others. I have sometimes seen a two-tier system, where English-speaking clients are interviewed by professionals with advanced degrees and a great deal of training, while Spanish-speaking clients are passed on to a professional who may be much less qualified in his or her field but speaks Spanish. Clearly, simply speaking Spanish (or Mandarin or Swahili) does *not* qualify a person to conduct a sensitive interview with a child any more than simply speaking English qualifies a person to do the work. Interviewers and therapists who conduct their work in a language other than English should have the same kind of training and supervision as everyone else. If the police officers who conduct child interviews in English have been trained in working with children, then the officers who conduct these interviews in languages other than English should be similarly trained.

When the child is interviewed in his or her first language only, the interviewer needs to have a clear plan about how to proceed. It is unrealistic to expect an interviewer to conduct an interview in Korean, for instance, and then simultaneously interpret everything into English for those watching behind the mirror. Rather, there should be a qualified interpreter behind the mirror to interpret for the observers, so the interviewer can concentrate on conducting the best possible interview.

Additionally, if the interview is conducted in a jurisdiction where video- or audiotapes are admissible in court, there needs to be a plan about how the documentation will be presented. Alternatives include transcribing the entire tape (or only important sections) and translating the transcription, putting English subtitles onto the tape, or having an interpreter describe what is being said in English in court. Each of these options has advantages and disadvantages, including cost. The prosecutors may choose to enter a summary of the evidence garnered during the interview rather than submitting the entire tape.

## Interviewing with an Interpreter

The third option for conducting interviews with nonnative speakers is using an interpreter. Please see Chapter 7 for more information on this topic.

## Bilingual Interviews

The fourth and final option for interviewing nonnative speakers is for a bilingual professional to conduct a bilingual interview, switching from one language to another as the child does. This professional will be able to understand the cultural issues and nuances in the conversation. In my opinion, this is clearly the best choice. All our agencies should employ qualified multilingual people whenever possible. Some bilingual children prefer to speak about their assault in the language in which it occurred. Others prefer to use a different language, to distance themselves from it. Still others will use both. Some bilingual children will say they are comfortable being interviewed in English, and will begin in this language. But as they enter the more emotionally laden content of the interview, they will begin responding in their native language, without even realizing it. A bilingual interviewer can follow the child's lead.

A bilingual, bicultural professional will be able to detect and interpret cultural cues as they emerge in an interview, and identify those concepts that cannot be easily translated from one culture to another. A bilingual professional can also more effectively communicate with the accompanying adults in cases where the children may speak English but their parents do not. It is not fair to ask children to interpret for their parents in this already stressful situation.

## Nonverbal Communication

### Gestures

Gestures have different meanings in different cultures and may be confusing. Many people use the gestures associated with their first language even when they are speaking English. Nonverbal cues can confuse an interviewer who is from a different culture.

For instance, an interviewer may ask a Latin American teenager a question, and the teenager responds with a shrug of the shoulders. The uninformed interviewer may assume that this gesture means "I don't know," whereas for many Latinos it means "I don't care" or "I don't want to talk about it," which is a very different message!

In court, an attorney may ask a child to point to the abuser, and expect the child to use his or her index finger. Among people from many Asian countries including China and the Philippines, it is impolite to point with a finger, and the child is apt to point with his or her chin and lips. Somali Bantus also consider it impolite to point to a person with the finger. Variations in nonverbal communication are endless and fascinating (see Axtell, 1998). In Chile, for instance, a wink signals assent. Of course, interviewers cannot learn all gestures for all cultures. But they should try to learn the gestures from the major ethnic groups in their catchment area—even if they work through interpreters.

The most important attribute for an interviewer in a cross-cultural encounter is a friendly and open attitude. If the interviewer is not sure what it means when a child winks or makes a hand gesture, he or she can rephrase the question or say, "I'm not sure what you mean. Can you explain that for me, please?" or "Can you give words to that?"

Male interviewers may need to be careful with their body posture, particularly with women and children from cultures different from their own. For instance, men should avoid sitting with their legs spread wide open, essentially exposing their genitals. When working with Muslims, they should avoid sitting with one leg over the other, exposing the sole of foot, which may be considered insulting. Additionally, large men should be mindful of how they use their size, positioning themselves in as nonthreatening a posture as possible. Male law enforcement officers may be accustomed to using their size to intimidate suspects. This would be inappropriate with a child or teenage victim, who needs reassurance, not intimidation.

## Seating Arrangements

Some guidelines recommend that interviewers sit across from the child, face to face. Many law enforcement officers habitually adopt this placement because it has been shown to work in offender interrogations. However, this positioning may seem unnaturally distant and confrontive to children from many cultures. I recommend that the interviewer and the child sit catty-corner, at the corner of a table, at a children's table, on comfortable chairs, or on the floor. This allows the child to face the interviewer when he or she wants, and avert eye contact when he or she desires more privacy.

## Eye Contact

White middle-class Anglo-Americans often expect children to look them in the eye when holding a conversation. In fact, some guidelines on interviewing children suggest that the interviewer maintain eye contact. However, children in many cultures have been taught that it is disrespectful to look adults in the eye. If an interviewer stares into a child's eyes and seeks out contact, the child may believe he or she is about to be punished. Interviewers should approach children in a friendly way, but not actively seek out eye contact. The presence or absence of eye contact should never be used as a gauge of truthfulness.

## Physical Expressiveness and Tone of Voice

People from different cultures vary in how much they move their eyebrows, foreheads, arms, and bodies while they speak. Interviewers need to be careful about how they view a child or adult who is either more or less physically expressive than they expect. Someone who is physically expressive may *seem* angry or theatrical, and someone who shows a still face may *seem* uncooperative or depressed. However, the person may just be acting in the way he or she learned to act in his or her culture. For example, Veronica Abney, an African American psychologist, describes being called down periodically to the emergency room of the hospital where she worked to help the White professionals handle Black mothers whom they said were "hysterical" (personal communication, 1998). She describes encountering mothers who are, naturally, upset because their children are in the emergency room, and who express their upset with stronger displays of emotion than the emergency room personnel are accustomed to seeing (e.g., by weeping, breathing deeply, sighing, calling out to God). Pathologizing this behavior by labeling it "hysterical" is not apt to be helpful. Conversely, sometimes Western professionals think Japanese parents are lying, depressed, or uncooperative because they tend to move their lips, eyebrows, and faces less than Westerners do in conversation (Axtell, 1998).

Tones of voice also vary with cultures. People from some cultures tend to speak loud, and people from other cultures more softly. The Chinese language is tonal. Chinese speakers are often perceived by English speakers to be angry because of the way they use their voices. Similarly, to people less familiar with the languages, speakers of Arabic, Vietnamese, and some African languages often sound like they are yelling angrily. An interviewer who is not accustomed to these language habits may find him- or herself responding to a Chinese parent as if he is angry, when he may not be. Puerto Ricans tend to vary their voice and speak in a sweet, singsong manner with children when they are not angry. Interviewers who speak in a steady monotone may be perceived by Puerto Rican children as unfriendly, hostile, and cold.

In cross-cultural encounters, professionals need to tune into their own responses. Sometimes when people are uncomfortable in a conversation but are not sure why, it is due to culturally based differences in nonverbal communication. It is important to avoid interpreting these crossed signals in a way that stigmatizes the child or his or her family.

## Touch

Some cultures rely more on touch than on words for comfort. When young children are upset during interviews, they sometimes want to hug or sit on the interviewer's lap. Of course this can happen with children from all cultural groups, but it may be especially common with children from cultures that tend to be physically close and demonstrative. Generally, interviewers should not have children sit on their laps during the interview—it is especially important to keep boundaries clear with children who may have had their boundaries violated. Interviewers can say, simply, "I see you want to be close to me. You can't sit in my lap, but why don't you pull your chair up right close to mine?"

Similarly, certain kinds of touch are problematic. For example, in Canada and the United States, adults frequently pat children on the head as a sign of affection, but this is a demeaning gesture for some Chinese, Filipino, and African American children, and the top of the head is considered a sacred spot and off-limits for casual touch by some Native Americans. People from certain religious groups, including some Muslims, Orthodox Jews, the Amish, and some conservative Christians, will not touch people of the opposite sex. The interviewer who extends his or her hand to shake the hand of a parent of the other sex may find that the hand is rejected. This should not be interpreted as a rejection of the interviewer's person.

## Pace and Silence

As much as possible, children should set the pace of the interview. Often children need more time to answer questions than one might expect. In my family growing up, if I did not interrupt someone, I could not get a word in edgewise; this is not an uncommon experience for people who come from large families or from cultural groups that value talkativeness. In many cultures, however, including many Native American and Asian cultures, long pauses between utterances are expected. Among the Inuit of Arctic, Quebec, mature children are expected to "control their tongues" and know when to stop talking (Crago, 1992). Intelligence is equated with quietness.

Middle-class American children from the majority group are usually encouraged to speak a lot. But Asian and Native American children, for example, may have been taught to choose their words carefully, to pause after questions, and to avoid speaking all the time, "like a fool." In Korea, for example, there is an expression that refers to big talkers, "The empty carriage makes a lot of noise" (Kim & Markus, 2002). The interviewer should strive to tune in to the child's own speaking rhythm.

Interviewers may need to learn to be comfortable with silence. Silence does not necessarily mean the child is about to lie, or needs help to come up with an answer. If the interviewer jumps in too quickly, trying to be helpful, the interviewer may actually make it more difficult for the child to speak.

## CLOSURE AND PREPARATION
## FOR THE NEXT STEPS

The interviewer may decide to end a conversation about child abuse because all the information has surfaced, because no information is forthcoming, because the time is up, or because the child needs to stop. The courts sometimes prefer a disclosure that happens all in one session. But children often cannot open up in one session—particularly those children who are suspicious of authorities. Disclosure is often a process, not a one-time event. Interviewers may need to schedule more than one interview (Carnes, 2000). Especially when interviews are stressful, interviewers need to save time at the end for children to regain their composure. Interviewers should close on a pleasant and supportive note. Children should be praised for speaking, and assured that they did the right thing. The interviewer should tell the child about the next steps in the process and allow the child to ask questions. Children—and particularly children who are less familiar with the workings of the child protection system in the United States—may have unrealistic ideas about the results of an interview (they may expect that the interviewer will take the child home with him or her, for instance, or will put him or her in jail).

Professionals cannot know the full impact of disclosing child abuse on a given child or family. In tightly knit Latino families, often a child who discloses is isolated from the rest of the family and barred from playing with his or her cousins. Essentially, he or she is ejected from the family. This may be experienced as a punishment close to torture, and will result in the child's recantation of the original disclosure if the child does not receive adequate support. Child abuse professionals in California have told me that Asian children who have disclosed are often pressured especially hard by their extended families to recant and sacrifice themselves so the family will not be destroyed and disgraced. These children and their nonoffending parents may need extra support and guidance. Interviewers may need to convey concerns in this regard to child protection workers, family advocates, police, and others.

## CONCLUDING THOUGHTS

The difficult and important process of interviewing a child or family about suspected maltreatment can become especially problematic when the interviewer and the child come from culturally distinct groups. In this chapter I have described several areas in which interviewers can adjust their practices to fit more appropriately with children from diverse cultural groups. I believe that interviewers can be successful with most children who differ from them culturally if they speak the same language, if the professional makes an effort to understand the child's culture, and if the professional demonstrates competence, caring, and trustworthiness.

### QUESTIONS TO THINK ABOUT AND DISCUSS

1. Have you ever conducted an interview where cultural differences seemed to get in the way? If so, please describe it.

2. How would you describe your professional identity to a nonoffending mother who is accompanying her child to an interview for suspected child abuse or neglect?

3. How would you describe the purpose of the interview to a 6-year-old child with limited English proficiency? And to a 12-year-old?

4. Think about a child from a particular ethnic minority group. Describe some of the special difficulties that child might face in the context of a forensic interview, and how you would overcome them if you were the interviewer.

5. Think about your own ethnic cultural background. How might this background affect the way you interview children (consider level of warmth, tone of voice, gestures, pace, etc.)? Is there anything you'd like to be able to adjust, according to the person you interview?

# CHAPTER FIVE

# Physical Discipline and Abuse

This chapter explores common areas of misunderstanding between professionals and cultural minority families around issues of discipline and physical abuse.[1] It presents research on corporal punishment and advocates for the elimination of all forms of violence toward children. I describe ways in which cultural practices including discipline can be misinterpreted as physical abuse, and offer reasons why minority families may be overinvestigated and reported for suspicions of physical abuse. I also discuss ways in which families' cultural values can be supported at the same time their harsh disciplinary practices can be challenged. Finally, I suggest ways to think about corporal punishment, discipline, and physical abuse that will maximize protection for all children, while minimizing harm to families.

Sue and James Johnson were African American professionals who lived in Springfield, Massachusetts, and raised their three children, ages 6–12, with a clear sense of right and wrong. The parents took their children to church regularly, prohibited their use of "street" language, and monitored their homework conscientiously. Much to their chagrin, when their eldest son, Derek, reached middle school he be-

---

[1]This chapter focuses on discipline and physical abuse in part because it is in the line between these two practices that cultural conflict often emerges. A thorough discussion of treatment for physical abuse is beyond the scope of this chapter. Several methods for working clinically with families to reduce physical abuse have been found to be helpful, including family therapy and individual cognitive behavioral therapy with parents (see Kolko, 1996) and parent child interaction therapy, which works with a parent–child dyad (see Borrego, Urquiza, Rasmussen, & Zebell, 1999). These methods and others have been found to be more effective than routine community-based services when working with diverse families where children have been abused physically. Each of these techniques can be adapted for maximum cultural competency, using the suggestions in this book.

came "wilder" and began hanging out with a rough crowd. When Derek came home with a report card full of poor grades, James struck him with a belt. Instead of crying as he had done in the past, Derek smirked while he was being beaten. His father responded by striking him harder than he had ever done before. In gym class the next day, Derek's teacher questioned him about the marks, and then called child protective services. An investigator interviewed Derek at school and then the parents and the other children at home. Based on the marks that were still visible, abuse charges against the parents were substantiated. The parents were asked to sign a treatment plan obligating them to attend parenting classes for 8 weeks and submit to periodic unannounced visits from a social worker. Sue and James were furious. They felt they did not need "some damn shrink" to tell them how to raise their children. They contended that the White social worker could not understand what it was like to raise a Black boy in a racist world, where his compliance with authority could be a question of life or death.

Is this a case of government do-gooders running riot with parents' efforts to raise their children properly? Is it a case of racist interference and lack of understanding of Black family values and social pressures? Or is it a case of the child welfare system stepping in to protect a vulnerable youngster, and his younger siblings, from well-meaning but abusive discipline? These are important questions to consider.

As I stated earlier, cultural minority children deserve the same protection from harsh physical punishment as White or mainstream children. Available research supports this position (McCord, 1996; Straus & Donnelly, 2001).[2] And yet the goal of protecting children from harsh corporal punishment is not easy to achieve in a culturally competent way.

When we work on issues of child discipline and physical abuse, we need to understand the systemic stresses that weigh upon many minority and low-income families, often contributing to disciplinary encounters and violence. If possible, we should look for helpful ways to reduce those stresses.

It is important to remember that individual members of a single cultural minority group vary widely in their acceptance and use of corporal punishment. For instance, although African Americans as a group have higher rates of corporal punishment today than White Americans (Ferrari, 2002), many African American parents disapprove of it and use *no* corpo-

---

[2]The literature is not unanimous but is, in my opinion, persuasive. Because this book is focused on practice rather than research, I will not discuss the literature in depth here, but refer readers to the work of Murray Straus.

ral punishment at all. Also, we should be aware that some studies have found higher rates of *physical abuse* among White families, as will be discussed below. Finally, in a wide variety of studies using vignettes to measure approval of harsh corporal punishment and physical abuse, Latinos, African Americans, Whites, and Asians show remarkable agreement in condemning abusive disciplinary practices (Maiter, Alaggia, & Trocmé, 2004; Ferrari, 2002). We should not make assumptions about a family's use of corporal punishment or the possible presence of physical abuse based on its group identity. Instead, we should inquire respectfully about what practices the members of a specific family believe in, and what they actually do.

Cultural minority parents who engage in physical abuse need help, but their needs are far from homogeneous. They fall into four major groups. In the first group, like the Johnson family discussed earlier, some are adequate or even excellent parents in other ways, and their authoritarian style and corporal punishment exist side by side with high levels of intimacy and support. (They may consider themselves practitioners of "tough love" or "old-fashioned discipline.") In these families corporal punishment may occasionally slip to levels that are considered abusive. The second group consists of members of religious minorities who are absolutely convinced of the rightness of physically abusive corporal punishment and other child-rearing practices that society considers dangerous. Sometimes these parents see such child-raising techniques as so central to their religious identity and mission that they are willing to go to jail, or even to allow their children to die, to meet their religious "obligation" (Swan, 1998). The third group encompasses parents who are struggling with issues of extreme poverty, mental illness, or substance abuse, and whose lives are filled with such chaos that they are considered neglectful as well as abusive. The fourth group comprises parents who punish their children in cruel and malicious ways that would be considered abusive in any culture. This chapter primarily pertains to the first group: those parents who mean well but rely on forms of punishment that are harsh and may sometimes become abusive. Unlike the other three groups, with these parents a culturally competent psychoeducational approach may be sufficient.

## RESEARCH ON GROUP DIFFERENCES

Some professionals may expect that immigrants and members of minority ethnic groups are more apt to be physically abusive toward their children than native-born White people. Research does not support this viewpoint (Maiter et al., 2004). However, it is difficult to make sense of all the many contradictions in the extensive literature on group differences in child physical abuse. Some of the confusion stems from the variety of methods used to gather data and variations in definitions. In 1985 the Children's Defense Fund issued a report stating that African American children are three times as likely to die from child abuse as White children. These differences are apt to be at least partially attributable to the poverty in which many Black families lived at the time (and continue to live) rather than to anything intrinsic to Black families—many of these children died of poverty-related neglect rather than physical abuse per se. Indeed, "Children from families earning an annual income below $15,000 were 22 times more likely to be abused than those from families earning $30,000 or more" (Kapp, McDonald, & Diamond, 2001, p. 216). Black children are almost four times as likely to be poor as White children (Federal Interagency Forum on Child and Family Statistics, 2004). Some have questioned the great disparity between Black and White deaths attributable to child abuse, wondering whether this difference stems partly from a bias in the classification of deaths rather than to their true causes, with perhaps a lack of willingness to classify the deaths of White children as homicides, and their deaths being classified as "accidental" or "of undetermined causes" instead (Sedlak, Bruce, & Schultz, 2001).

While some studies have found that African American children are more at risk for physical abuse than White children (e.g., Connelly & Straus, 1992), others have found that African American children were *less* likely to be maltreated by their *mothers* than White children (e.g., Zuravin, 1989). This would suggest that African American children may be at risk due to their increased exposure to caretakers *other than* their mothers. Indeed, it has been found that White children are more likely to be abused by a biological parent, whereas non-White children are more likely to be abused by someone other than a parent or parent substitute (as cited in Kapp et al., 2001). Additionally, we must remember that social class and race are highly correlated in North America, and this may influence all racial data on child maltreatment.

Ferrari (2002) examined the idea that parental cultural *values* rather than parental ethnicity per se would place children at risk or protect them from physical abuse. Indeed, she found that fathers of all ethnicities who valued *familism* (a close-knit family) were less likely to use physical punishment, and fathers who valued *machismo* (defined loosely as adhering to rigid sex roles and male dominance) were more likely to use physical punishment and less likely to show nurturance with their sons. Ferrari found few ethnic differences in the ratings of child abuse and neglect vignettes, suggesting that increased rates of reports to child protective services and involvement with the child welfare system "cannot be attributed to society's lack of a culturally specific definition of child maltreatment" (p. 809). Ferrari found that African American mothers did use more physical and verbal punishment than other mothers in the sample, but also were higher in nurturing behaviors, which may buffer some of the potential negative effects of physical punishment. This is just a sample of the muddle of complicated findings that concern racial and cultural differences in attitudes and practices related to physical punishment, physical abuse, and child welfare involvement in diverse families. Much remains to be known about the interplays of poverty, education, culture, family configuration, stress, availability of childcare, and so on in increasing or decreasing a child's risk of being subject to physical abuse. Much also remains to be known about the interplays of racism; an inadequate social support net; lack of access to quality healthcare, housing, and schools; and professional bias in the racial disparity in family involvement in child welfare.

In a sense, the relative percentage of physical abuse among different groups does not really matter. We know that physical abuse occurs within *some* families in *all* groups, and should be reduced. This chapter focuses on members of cultural minority groups *not* because they might be at higher risk for physical abuse, but rather because (1) preventive efforts are more likely to be effective if they are tailored to the needs of the group they are meant to address; (2) professionals frequently insult and therefore alienate cultural minority parents when they discuss concerns about disciplinary techniques and raise the specter of abuse; and (3) professionals are often puzzled about how to handle families' right to punish children in a way that fits with their culture and values, while at the same time protecting the youngsters. I cannot provide definitive answers for working with *all* cultural minority families. Rather, I discuss recent research on corporal punishment, call attention to cultural issues regarding the line between physical punishment and abuse, and provide general guidelines for working with cultural minority families whose punishment techniques appear harsh.

## CORPORAL PUNISHMENT AND PHYSICAL ABUSE

### Definitions and Data

Straus and Donnelly (2001) define corporal punishment as "the use of physical force with the intention of causing a child to experience pain, but not injury, for the purpose of correction or control of the child's behavior" (p. 4). Some public health advocates have described corporal punishment more critically as "a form of intrafamilial violence associated with short and long-term adverse mental health outcomes" (Stewart et al., 2000, p. 257). Corporal punishment in the United States presents a complex picture, with high but decreasing rates of general approval, and a population increasingly divided in regard to its use (Straus & Donnelly, 2001; Straus & Mathur, 1994). Public approval of corporal punishment in the United

States decreased dramatically from 94% in 1968 to 68% in 1994 (Straus, 2001; Straus & Mathur, 1996). In 1968 there was almost universal approval in the United States for parents spanking children, regardless of demographic variables. But by 1994 the picture had become more complex. Corporal punishment is currently most heavily supported by African Americans, Southerners, and people with fewer years of formal education (Straus & Donnelly, 2001; Straus & Mathur, 1996).

In 1998, the American Academy of Pediatrics's official policy statement on effective discipline included the following assertions:

> Corporal punishment is of limited effectiveness and has potentially deleterious side effects. The American Academy of Pediatrics recommends that parents be encouraged and assisted in the development of methods other than spanking for managing undesired behavior. . . . Other forms of physical punishment, such as striking a child with an object, striking a child on parts of the body other than the buttocks or extremities, striking a child with such intensity that marks lasting more than a few minutes occur, pulling a child's hair, jerking a child by the arm, shaking a child, and physical punishment delivered in anger with intent to cause pain, are unacceptable and may be dangerous to the health and well-being of the child. These types of physical punishment should never be used.[3] (pp. 723, 726)

The actual *use* of corporal punishment in the United States is also decreasing, along with public approval of it (Daro & Gelles, 1992; Straus & Donnelly, 2001). Even so, corporal punishment is still used widely.

Unfortunately, data concerning immigrants is limited. Frequently, immigrants are simply excluded from the sample, or are miscoded as African American, White, or "other," categories that reveal little about differences among people of various national origins. Maiter et al. (2004) have begun filling this gap with information on South Asian families in Canada.

Data on the use of corporal punishment among people of various religious groups is also limited (Bottoms & Shaver, 1995). In most big cities the media have reported on members of small religious groups defending their use of abusive and sometimes fatal corporal punishment on religious grounds. In 2001, for example, the House of Prayer in Atlanta, Georgia, a church with some 150 members, was found to condone the beating of children with belts and switches (as well as the marriage of girls as young as 14). In fact, the pastor often helped restrain the children and supervised the beatings. The police found open wounds and three-inch-long welts on children (Firestone, 2001). These claims to "religious freedom" have met with varying degrees of success in the courts (Johnson, 1998). Levesque (2001) writes:

---

[3]Canadian pediatric societies have issued similar statements (Durrant, Ensom, & the Coalition on Physical Punishment of Children and Youth, 2004).

The United States already is home to many forms of abuse that continue partly because of religious protections. A most notable example involves the corporal punishment of children. Although increasingly challenged, a main rationale that permits the corporal punishment of children is the religious conviction that directs parents to use force. The rise in religious fundamentalism seeks legal reform, which not only would protect parents who inflict violence but also create environments that several researchers view as conducive to family violence. (p. 80)

Put simply, although the U.S. public as a whole increasingly disapproves of corporal punishment, as evidenced by the response of the general public and influential groups such as pediatricians, this trend coexists with extensive continued use of corporal punishment and efforts by some groups to assert a legal right to punish their children physically in ways that are currently considered abusive.

## Drawing the Line

Where do we draw the line between corporal punishment and physical abuse? Graziano (1994) hypothesizes a continuum, ranging from low to high violence. On one end of the spectrum are extremely violent acts that almost anyone would agree constitute physical abuse, such as those resulting in permanent injury or death. On the other end of the spectrum are those actions that most people do *not* consider abusive, such as a gentle slap to a toddler's hand when the toddler reaches for a hot stove.

[However], the central portion of this spectrum, where accepted discipline begins to shade into abuse, does not carry a standard definition by which all of us would agree on exactly where acceptable discipline becomes abuse. What is deemed acceptable by some will be considered abusive by others. (Graziano, 1994, p. 415)

In most areas state law is of little help in demarcating the line between corporal punishment and physical abuse, since the language used, such as "leaving a mark" or "resulting in physical or psychological damage," leaves wide room for interpretation. In this chapter, I refer to the problematic middle of this spectrum of behaviors as "harsh physical punishment," knowing that even this term is open to question, since any two individuals could easily debate about what is "harsh." (When working with parents who have engaged in abusive discipline, it can be helpful to use the words "discipline" or "punishment" rather than "abuse" to avoid engaging in a battle around whether a particular action falls into the category of "abuse.")

It is important to note the connection between the two ends of the spectrum, corporal punishment and physical abuse. Straus and Donnelly (2001) define physical abuse as any "attack on a child that results in an injury" (p. 9). Most episodes of physical abuse begin as disciplinary encounters. That is, a parent or other caretaker uses corporal punishment with the intention of punishing a child, teaching a child a lesson, or correcting a child's misbehavior, but the child is injured because of an accident or excessive use of force. The case of the Johnson family falls into this category. In another, more tragic example, a mother intended to slap her 6-year-old daughter Lucía across the face, but Lucía turned her head and the mother's fingernail slashed her eye and damaged her retina. The mother was so afraid of the authorities that she failed to seek medical care, and the daughter ended up blind in one eye. This was a case of corporal punishment that resulted in permanent injury, and therefore can be classified as physical abuse. Unfortunately, cases of corporal punishment that somehow cross the line into abuse are all too common. Many a parent can be heard weeping in hospital emergency rooms, "I didn't mean to *hurt* him!"

Routine use of corporal punishment leads too many parents to inflict physical abuse on their children because milder forms of corporal punishment lose their effectiveness over time, and because the parents' reliance on physical methods of control results in a decreased ability to control the children through nonphysical means (Graziano, 1994; McCord, 1996). Also, the higher the number of disciplinary encounters, the more likely it is that a child will be abused (Straus & Donnelly, 2001). Reducing the number of disciplinary incidents and eliminating corporal punishment are important first steps to eliminating physical abuse in a family. Put simply, if I never strike my children, there is no possibility that I will strike them too hard.

Although research shows that family stress contributes to a greater likelihood of physical abuse, it is unclear which specific stressors are most important as causes of abuse among families from diverse cultural groups. Cultural and familial factors may mitigate certain stressors. For example, while children who live in crowded quarters generally suffer from higher levels of physical abuse, research on Arabs, African Americans, and Latinos suggest that this may be less true if the cohabitants are members of an extended family (Ferrari, 2002; Youssef, Attia, & Kamel, 1998). The presence of a grandmother, in particular, appears to be associated with a more responsive and less punitive parenting style among African American and Latino families (García Coll, 1990). In studies among mixed populations, the following stressors have been correlated with physical child abuse: paternal unemployment, poverty, single-parent families, parental substance abuse, adult mental health problems, social isolation, neighborhood deterioration, and—importantly—physical abuse of the mother by the father.

There are higher rates of child physical abuse by both mothers and fathers in families where the father is physically violent toward the mother (Edleson, 1999).

As a corollary to these findings, to reduce levels of physical child abuse we must help parents (1) reduce the number and severity of disciplinary encounters with their children; (2) reduce or eliminate their use of corporal punishment; (3) reduce parental isolation and stress; and (4) detect and eliminate the battering of women. Professionals must be sure to engage in these strategies in culturally competent ways.

## CULTURE IN DISCIPLINE AND ABUSE

In the last few years a number of social scientists and mental health practitioners have begun to explore connections between physical abuse, discipline, and culture (e.g., DeYoung & Zigler, 1994; Ferrari, 2002; Fontes, 2000). These works typically concern African American parents (see Bradley, 1998) and fundamentalist Christian parents (e.g., Swan, 1998). Research on immigrant parents is limited (e.g., Maiter et al., 2004; Negroni, 1998; Zayas & Solari, 1994).

Child rearing is highly influenced by ethnic culture. What children need to learn, and the methods considered best for teaching them, are passed down from one generation to another as cultural knowledge and tradition. Norms around acceptable child rearing and punishment vary by culture. For example, in the Pacific Island nation of Palau, parents commonly tie the leg of a toddler to a post or door with a rope when the parents are unable to supervise the child directly, such as when they are out farming. In Palau, parents also commonly spank children with a broom, breaking the skin and leaving bruises, when the children do not do their chores or homework (Collier, McClure, Collier, Otto, & Polloi, 1999). While these practices would be considered abusive in the U.S. and Canada, some people from other cultures might see abuse in the common U.S. practices of circumcising male infants, denying children food between mealtimes, washing children's mouths out with soap, or forcing infants to cry themselves to sleep at night alone (Korbin & Spilsbury, 1999).

Cultural subgroups within the United States and Canada also vary widely in the methods they use to enforce discipline and gain compliance. In a fascinating article about a discussion on discipline held by elderly African American women, Mosby, Rawls, Meehan, Mays, and Pettinori (1999) describe the older women's preference for a "light tap" or a "touch" with a hand or a switch, delivered without anger at the moment of the transgression, over cursing or screaming at a child, which they deemed a form of child abuse.

Studies have reported that African Americans and people from the southern United States and the Caribbean are more likely to punish their children with an electric cord, belt, or switch applied to the back or bottom (Payne, 1989; Showers & Bandman, 1986). European (White) Americans are more likely to use a paddle or an open hand to the bottom. Recent Korean immigrants may slap a child's face and pull the child's hair. Chinese parents may pinch their youngsters more than other parents do. And Puerto Rican families may place a toddler who is having a tantrum into a bathtub of cold water.

Many families have an item available at hand that they use in a habitual way to punish a child, and this punishment may reach abusive levels. Examples that I have encountered include:

- Objects that a child is made to kneel on with bare knees for minutes or hours, such as an abacus (Chinese families), a tray of uncooked rice (Latino and Asian families), uncooked grains of corn (Central American families), gravel (families from some parts of Africa), salt (Jamaican families), or a cheese grater or heating grate (U.S. families).
- Matching Bibles that the child is forced to hold out in his or her hands with arms extended (fundamentalist Christians).
- Potions that the child is forced to drink that work as laxatives or make him or her vomit.
- Soap that is used to "wash out" the mouth of a child who has cursed.
- A special jar of pepper that can be rubbed in the child's eyes or genitals.
- A jar of hot peppers that the child is forced to eat when he or she says something wrong.
- A whip, belt, electric cord, strap, paddle, or wooden switch that is used to administer thrashings. This object may have a special name, such as "the Doctor" or "Mr. Trouble."
- A "prayer" closet where a child is locked up in darkness to contemplate what he or she has done wrong.

Unfortunately, the list of instruments that people use against their children is endless. While cultural differences influence the *kinds* of physical discipline used, they do not determine whether these punishments constitute abuse in any given instance, since each one of these methods can be applied gently or with great force, frequently or rarely, for a long or a short duration. Additionally, Ferrari's work (2002) suggests that although there are ethnic differences in the use of corporal punishment, there is great agreement on when that punishment crosses the line into abuse.

Sometimes culturally based punishments involve a symbolic element. Here I will give examples from Latino families—but these kinds of examples exist for members of other groups as well. A child who curses may be slapped across the mouth (a *tapaboca*). A child who has done or said something considered stupid may be knuckled on the top of the head (a *cocotazo*). A child who has been disrespectful may be made to kneel on uncooked rice or corn with bare knees (*hincar*). A child who has stolen something may have his or her hands slapped. Parents may place pepper in the eyes of a teenager who has trouble waking up in the morning and is consistently late to school or work; or place pepper on the genitals of a child who masturbates. With the exception of the last two examples, whether these punishments constitute physical abuse depends on their severity, how often they are used, and their effect on the children. (Pepper can damage sensitive tissues, and children have died from aspirating pepper that they were being forced to eat as a punishment [Socolar & Runyan, 2001].)

Why do cultures vary in the ways they choose to discipline and punish their children? There are numerous reasons. Parents punish their children in order to teach them the behaviors that will be most helpful within the context of the society in which they are growing up. Other differences may stem from the objects that are available at hand in a particular physical environment to inflict the punishment. Religious ideas about sin, purity, and redemption undoubtedly influence parents' attitudes toward punishment. If a religion teaches that children are born with a good nature that requires nurturing, they are apt to be treated more gently than if they are believed to be born with an evil nature that needs to be broken and bent toward righteousness. Children born into cultures that were once victimized by colonialism and/or slavery are often treated especially harshly: the parents have inherited a cultural tradition that prepared them to face the harshness of their master's or colonizer's rule. The harsh punishments may be inflicted with love and with the intention of keeping the children safe from a harsh world, but the punishments may nevertheless be dangerous.

## CHILD-RAISING NORMS

Traditionally oriented families may be more likely to employ an authoritarian style of parenting and to demand obedience and respect from their children. These practices clash with the child-rearing norms of the dominant culture, which tend to tolerate back-talk, foster independence, and emphasize peer rather than family connections. Cultures vary in how much they value children's opinions and needs, and the importance they give to childhood as a separate phase of life. They also vary in their assessment of the best way to care for children. For example, Mexican infants and toddlers

tend to be held by adults throughout the day and are rarely given opportunities to crawl. Mexican infants and toddlers tend to be clothed heavily even
in hot temperatures, to protect them from the elements. Their parents tend
to feed them with a bottle or spoon through their toddler years, rather than
allowing them to self-feed messily. Mexican children often sleep with their
parents until age 6 or older, or until another child is born who takes their
place in the parental bed. Some Mexican families view U.S. culture as
remarkably unfriendly to children.

By comparison, Anglo-American infants and toddlers in the United
States and Canada are often placed on a blanket or carpet or on the floor
during the day so they can build strength and independence. They are encouraged to crawl and explore the world on their own. Their parents give
them opportunities to self-feed before a year of age, and photographs of
infants with cereal smeared over their face and hair grace many family al-
bums. (A child who was dirty with food in this way would seem neglected
and unhygienic to many Mexican parents.) Anglo-American parents often
expect their infants to sleep alone from birth. Neither approach to child
rearing is necessarily preferable to the other. Rather, each shapes children
with personalities to fit their specific cultures.

Many cultures do not make as sharp a separation between the adult
and the child worlds, allowing children to attend family and neighborhood
events that occur late at night, and expecting children to entertain themselves in close proximity to adults, rather than separating them into camps
or children's play rooms. In addition, in many cultures children are cared
for by the collective community, rather than considered the sole property
of and responsibility of their parents. U.S. writer Barbara Kingsolver
(1995) described her experiences living with her 4-year-old daughter in the
Canary Islands of Spain:

> Widows in black, buttoned-down CEOs, purple-sneakered teenagers, the
> butcher, the baker, all would stop on the street to have little chats with my
> daughter. . . . Whenever Camille grew cranky in a restaurant (and really,
> what do you expect at midnight?) the waiters flirted and brought her little
> presents, and nearby diners looked on with that sweet, wistful gleam of an eye
> that I'd thought diners reserved for the dessert tray. What I discovered in
> Spain was a culture that held children to be its meringues and éclairs. My own
> culture, it seemed to me in retrospect, tended to regard children as a sort of
> toxic-waste product: a necessary evil, maybe, but if it's not our own we don't
> want to see it or hear it or, God help us, smell it. (p. 100)

Kingsolver discovered a society that accepted children's presence across a
wide variety of contexts and collectively contributed to the children's
well-being. In cultures where children are not tucked away into the privat-

ized sphere of the home, children may be punished in public in a way that puts the family at risk for reports of child maltreatment.

Some Asian immigrant families consider instilling discipline and obedience in their children their foremost duty, followed by enforcing academic success. Asian parents will sometimes severely restrict their children's activities during the school week to ensure that they have enough time to study and to sleep well. If they don't believe the schools are assigning sufficient homework, they may make devise additional homework assignments or problems for their children to complete.

## Punishing in Public

Members of cultural minority groups often feel that their behavior is viewed in a constant unforgiving spotlight. They feel pressured to appear as a model minority to counter prejudices against their group. For example, African Americans are often hesitant to leave their homes in very casual clothing to avoid supporting stereotypes of their group as unsuccessful or poor. Bad behavior on the part of one member of the group is perceived as reflecting on all. For example, when Woody Allen was accused of sexual abuse and O. J. Simpson was accused of murdering his wife, many Jews and African Americans, respectively, felt themselves to be on the defensive. The same pressure did *not* fall upon White Anglo-Saxon Protestants when Timothy McVeigh was found to be responsible for the Oklahoma City bombing, or when White boys engaged in mass school killings. Members of the dominant group who commit crimes are seen as individuals, whereas members of minority groups who commit crimes are seen as reflecting their entire group.

For this reason, many ethnic and religious minority parents consider it highly important that their children be well behaved and represent their family and culture well in public. Unlike many Anglo-American parents, who prefer to present a conflict-free public image, when parents who are members of visible minority groups see their children acting disobediently or disrespectfully in public, they are likely to punish them immediately and in public—placing them at greater risk for reports to child protection authorities. In the discussion group of elderly African American women described earlier, one participant emphasized the importance of stopping a child "right there" when he misbehaves, and the other women in the group agreed (Mosby et al., 1999): "She argued that the speedy use of physical discipline solves the problem quickly and prevents the slow build up of anger that leads to abuse" (p. 501). So while the woman's intention was to offer a rapid, appropriate response, and thus avoid abuse, the public nature of the response might place her at increased risk of involvement with child protection authorities.

# INTERVENING WITH FAMILIES WHO USE HARSH CORPORAL PUNISHMENT

We should be careful to distinguish between a single episode of physical abuse by caring parents that stems from acceptable discipline gone awry (e.g., a parent who grabbed a child too hard and left a mark on the arm) and intentional, repeated abuse in which physical and psychological damage is evident. Both need to be taken seriously and reported to protective services where indicated. But in the first case, education and stress reduction are probably the most appropriate remedies. In the second case, the parent may be evidencing severe psychological disturbance, substance abuse problems, or an actual dislike of the child. These factors must be resolved through more extensive interventions before skills training can prove beneficial.

Frequently, concerns about discipline emerge long before a reportable incident is suspected or revealed. This opens a window for preventing child abuse and averting intrusive interventions (see Chapter 8). When professionals are uncertain whether a given incident raises enough concern about physical abuse to file a report, they should consult with a colleague or supervisor. In addition, in most areas professionals can call their state protective service agency, describe the case without revealing the clients' names, and ask for advice. The intake workers often make an assessment as to whether the behaviors are sufficiently indicative of abuse to merit filing a report. Also, intake workers may indicate the kinds of additional information they would need before deciding to investigate a given family (see Chapter 3).

If the caretakers' disciplinary methods constitute physical abuse as defined by state law, and you become aware of an abusive episode through the course of your professional duties, or consider the child at risk, you are legally obliged to file a report with child protective services or the police. This holds true regardless of the family's cultural background. In my opinion, filing a report *without a family's knowledge* is apt to increase their feelings of isolation and mistrust and should be done only *when absolutely necessary to protect the child's immediate safety.* Rather, usually we *should try to file with protective services in a collaborative way* by explaining to the caretakers our legal obligations and letting the caretakers remain in the room during the phone call to protective services. In this way, the caretakers hear exactly what is being said about them. Many cultural minority families hold a deep distrust of professionals and authorities. Keeping caretakers in the loop early by telling them of our concerns can help us maintain a relationship with the family.

There will be occasions when a professional—using his or her judgment—will decide to file without informing the family first. Most state child protective service authorities will make an effort to keep the identity of the person who filed secret. However, one of two things often happens: either the family figures out the identity of the person who filed because of the kind of information held by protective services, or the family becomes mistrusting of all the professionals in their circle (physicians, teachers, counselors, etc.). In general, if I have a choice between having a family resent me and become angry at me, or having them resent and fear all professionals in their sphere, I'd rather take the heat.

Depending on the severity of the situation, resources available, and a host of other factors, protective services may choose not to investigate, may investigate and substantiate that abuse has occurred and close the case, or may investigate but then allow the family to proceed in their work with a counselor or therapist, avoiding foster care and other extreme interventions. In the great majority of cases, when a charge of child abuse or neglect is substantiated the case is readily closed without the provision of further services, because the agencies simply do not have the resources to provide ongoing supervision or psychotherapy to the vast numbers of families who have been found to have abused or neglected a child (Melton, 2003). This being true, professionals who work with families should know that our responsibilities related to child maltreatment do *not* begin and end with decisions about whether to report. If we hope to make a true difference in the lives of vulnerable families, our commitment and engagement must be more long term.

Professionals in many settings wonder what to do about situations where discipline seems harsh but does not cross into the illegal category of physical abuse, or where child protection authorities do not consider an incident sufficiently severe to intervene. After we have fulfilled our legal and ethical obligations in such cases, we still face a moral question as to how to proceed.

In the United States and Canada, parents do have a legal right to use corporal punishment with their children. Therefore, if we see our job as eliminating physical abuse only, then we might want to advise parents on how to punish their children gently without being culpable of physical abuse—for instance, by using one strike with an open hand on a clothed bottom only, and not engaging in this spanking while angry or more often than once a day.[3]

---

[3]Perhaps it is worth explaining why this method is considered preferable over others. With an open hand, the person who is administering the punishment is better able to feel the force of the hit, and therefore may be less likely to strike too hard. Also, striking the bottom allows some of the force to be absorbed by the fleshy buttocks, causing less trauma to internal organs. And, finally, the buttocks are not in close proximity to highly vulnerable organs, such as the eyes, brain, or kidneys. That said, children have been *killed* by their caretaker striking a buttock with an open hand with too much force (Lambert, 2002). Parents who have *ever* lost control and inflicted abuse while punishing should eliminate corporal punishment altogether).

As stated earlier, we should remember that the use of even mild forms of corporal punishment leads to an increased likelihood of physical abuse. Whatever suggestions are made to the parents in an attempt to find ways to discipline a child without committing abuse, there may be serious long-term drawbacks to using even mild forms of corporal punishment.

Even those forms of corporal punishment that do not qualify as illegal physical abuse have been correlated with a variety of negative outcomes for children (Straus & Donnelly, 2001), including higher rates of delinquency and aggression at school, and lower levels of academic and professional achievement. Therefore, I join the American Academy of Pediatrics in the belief that professionals have an obligation to work toward the elimination of corporal punishment, which will eliminate its potential harm. This obligation is particularly important, I believe, when considering minority children who already face discrimination, higher rates of poverty, and other obstacles. If we fail to address issues of corporal punishment among minority families because of a fear of imposing dominant norms on oppressed people, we leave minority children at increased potential risk.

## Building Opposition to Corporal Punishment

When people immigrate to the United States and Canada, they are obliged to adjust to their host society in myriad ways. Some they enjoy, and others they resent. For example, they may now have to live in a cold climate although they would prefer a warm one. They may be forced to speak English, although they might prefer to continue speaking their first language. Similarly, some parents might prefer to use punishment techniques that are considered abusive or harsh in their new country, but were acceptable "back home." However, we can sometimes persuade them to stop by citing the *appearance of abuse* this produces among their children's friends and among professionals including school personnel, and the negative ways this could impact upon the family. Parents also may decide to forgo corporal punishment when they are given information about recent research concerning its potential harmful effect on their children (e.g., Straus & Donnelly, 2001). At this point, a reader might wonder, "Does this position amount to pressure by professionals on families to acculturate, or is it sound advice?" Given that corporal punishment has *never* been found to benefit children more than *attentive parenting without it*, and that avoiding corporal punishment reduces the likelihood of disruptive child protection interventions, I believe it is sound advice. Further, the advice can be presented in ways that build upon desirable family strengths, such as loyalty, cohesiveness, and respect.

Firm discipline is deeply rooted in many African American families and institutions (Bradley, 1998). This tradition runs so deep that some parents feel as if they are turning their back on their ancestors and even on their race if they abandon corporal punishment. One scholarly article on physical discipline in African American families argued, "The right to raise one's children according to traditional beliefs should be as sacred under the constitution as the right to one's religious beliefs" (Mosby et al., 1999, p. 515). The pastor of the Atlanta, Georgia, church, House of Prayer, described above for the way he helped parents abusively assault their children and teenagers, was quoted as saying, "If the white society doesn't want to whip their children, that's their business. I'm not trying to make you black, so don't try to make me white" (Firestone, 2001, p. A14). Clearly, efforts by professionals representing mainstream institutions to reduce the use of corporal punishment can encounter great resistance in some communities (see Chapter 8).

However, other African Americans believe that physical punishment is a residue of slavery, and contributes to aggression among African American children (Vanderhorst, 1996; Hines & Boyd-Franklin, 1996). When working with African Americans, professionals of all backgrounds need to keep in mind the issues of loyalty to family and people, and the pressures of racism. A reassurance like the following may help:

> "It's hard for many parents to think about abandoning corporal punishment because they feel like they're being asked to reject the way their own parents raised them. Let me tell you right off that I am not questioning the way you were raised or criticizing *your* parents. Rather, I'm going to do my best to help you interact with your children in this day and age—which might require a different approach from the one that was used with us when we were children. In addition, whether you agree or disagree, if you use harsh corporal punishment with your children you run the risk of getting investigated by child protective services and getting your children taken away from you."

Parents who were raised with corporal punishment can often be heard saying things like "My parents gave me the strap and I turned out okay." To this I reply, "Probably you turned out okay because of what they were *doing* and *saying* before and after they strapped you. They spoke to you about the difference between right and wrong and set clear limits. I don't think it was the strapping itself that made you who you are." Parents of various ethnic groups usually agree.

Sometimes I also use a *smoking analogy* (Straus & Donnelly, 2001). Although not all cigarette smokers die of smoking-related illnesses, many do; and others may have more minor health problems (e.g., a chronic cough and shortness of breath) resulting from the smoking. No one would say that smoking is harmless because not everyone who smokes suffers the most severe outcome. Similarly, not all people who were punished physically become suicidal or end up in jail. Some do, however; and others suffer more subtle harm such as depression or impaired relationships. Since no benefit has been shown to derive from corporal punishment as compared to a loving, attentive parenting approach without it, then corporal punishment should be eliminated.

Professionals often wonder how to help parents abandon harsh corporal punishment. One option is to explain the laws and inform parents of the implications of their continued actions (e.g., "If you do not stop leaving bruises on your children, protective services might take away your children and you might end up in jail"). This seems to be the approach taken by most child protective service professionals. However, it is likely to be helpful only to those parents who were previously unaware of the laws and their implications, such as some immigrant parents. A second option is to help parents consider carefully the results of their actions. For example, professionals can ask parents the following questions: "Does this kind of punishment produce the results you want? How do you feel when you hit your child? Are you tired of punishing? Ideally, how often would you like to hit your child?" Some parents respond well to questions that help them tune in to their children's responses, such as "What does your child think and feel while being spanked?"

Upon questioning, many parents will readily admit that as time goes on they find themselves using corporal punishment more often and hitting harder than in the past. A frustrated parent who is asked "If there was a more effective method of discipline, would you use it?," will often respond affirmatively, opening the door for skill building (Fontes, 2002).

When asked what lesson a child learns from being spanked for lying, for instance, some caretakers will say that the child learns not to lie. Upon probing, however, they may admit that the child truly learns *not to get caught* lying. For the child to learn not to lie, the caretaker must discuss with the child the implications of lying and how lying can be hurtful. The physical punishment itself merely teaches the consequences for being caught, not the consequences for the misdeed itself. Of course, the child has also learned the hidden lesson of corporal punishment, which is that force or violence is the correct way to resolve difficulties.

## Creating New Meanings

Families who repeatedly use abusive corporal punishment are families who live by a story in which this is part of who they are and what they do. Parents will say "I believe in the stick, not the carrot" or "Sammy is hard-headed and he won't listen without a beating." This buy-in to corporal punishment as part of their identity reminds me of the person who smokes and says with a shrug, after seeing evidence of the harmfulness of smoking, "But I'm a smoker." Parents need to be invited into a new story of themselves as a family that is questioning—or actively abandoning—physical discipline. Sometimes parents who are helped to believe in the rightness of child rearing without violence are able to take this important step even without further skills training. Marcia, an African American participant in a workshop, spoke movingly about the time when she was spanking her 8-year-old daughter for misbehavior and the child turned to her and said simply, "Why don't you just talk to me instead of hitting me?" Marcia says she never raised her hand to her children again because she had suddenly stopped believing in it.

A fascinating piece of research on African American and White American mothers from a variety of social classes who decided to give up corporal punishment reveals that "although reasons for quitting vary, cessation is generally associated with new meanings that turn old beliefs into excuses and that define nonspanking as progress" (Davis, 1999, p. 492). Davis goes on to suggest that cultural inducements and social support may be as important as learning new disciplinary techniques.

Another fascinating study found that even among highly stressed parents, those who believed in corporal punishment showed greater potential for physically abusing their children than similarly stressed parents who did *not* believe in corporal punishment (Crouch & Behl, 2001). This finding underscores the importance of changing *ideas* about corporal punishment, as well as reducing stress, to reduce child abuse potential in parents.

Professionals can suggest that eliminating corporal punishment is *an ideal to work toward*, an ideal that some families achieve immediately by simply eliminating it from their vocabulary of behaviors, and that other families begin to achieve by significantly *reducing* its use. The next section suggests ways to invite caretakers to reconsider their use of corporal punishment by tapping into their best wishes for their children.

## Using Values to Motivate Change

## Ambition

Parents' ambitions for their children may be a source of motivation for the abandonment of corporal punishment. You can say something like:

> "Ways to encourage 'good behavior' that are not based on punishment are more likely to result in your children thinking for themselves, rather than depending on other people telling them what to do. If you teach them without hitting them, your children are more likely to

achieve better grades, get better jobs, and be more economically successful."

Most parents want their children to grow up safely, get rewarding jobs, be caring family members and decent people who make their parents proud. When working with a family, it is important to address these motivations directly by tapping into parents' noble intentions. Many members of cultural minority groups in the United States and Canada come from countries with recent histories of slavery and colonization. In these past circumstances, parents were probably saving their children's lives by teaching them how to obey authorities without question. We can safely assume, however, that few parents hope their children will grow up to hold the menial jobs where this kind of abject obedience might be valued (Payne, 1989). Rather, they hope their children will grow up to hold jobs where they will think for themselves, initiate ideas, and eventually supervise others. Professionals can inform and explore with parents the concept that children need to have an internalized sense of values to achieve these higher status positions, and that nonviolent methods of child raising teach children how to think and reason, not merely to avoid punishment. Additionally, parents may be impressed with the research showing that frequent use of corporal punishment reduces the likelihood of upward social mobility (Straus & Donnelly, 2001; Straus & Mathur, 1996), and has been associated with lower economic achievement in adulthood (Straus & Donnelly, 2001).

## School Success

Some parents will say they use corporal punishment so their children will learn to obey rules and avoid trouble in school. They are likely to be surprised by research showing that children who are punished corporally at home are *more* likely to be aggressive with their classmates (Straus & Donnelly, 2001; Strassberg, Dodge, Pettit, & Bates, 1994), and more likely to engage in delinquent and criminal behavior in their childhood. Recent research shows that corporal punishment actually increased the misbehaviors—it is not simply a question of adults being more likely to punish misbehaving youngsters (Straus & Donnelly, 2001).

It can be helpful to discuss this research with parents, and explain to them that when they are physically forceful with their children they are *modeling* the notion that physical force is the way to get what one wants. To explain the importance of modeling in educating children, you can mention examples that are not related to violence but would be familiar to the parents. For example, you might speak about how when we want a child to learn a given behavior—from tying shoes to cooking to using a hammer—we usually demonstrate it first, and the children copy what we do. By hitting, parents are inadvertently teaching children to hit others to get their way. Hitting children is a way of inadvertently teaching them that it is okay to give pain to others (McCord, 1996), and to use physical force when we really want something. Children who obey their parents because of the fear or threat of physical punishment may have a more difficult time obeying educators who do not hold this threat over their heads.

## Aggression and Delinquency

Sometimes parents, and particularly African American parents, will say that they especially need to use corporal punishment with their sons so that their sons will avoid getting tangled up in an unfair and discriminatory criminal justice system. Or—as some parents will say more plainly—"It's better that I whip him at home than that he gets shot by the police." These parents may be surprised to learn that corporal punishment actually *increases* the likelihood of children displaying aggressive, delinquent, and oppositional behavior (Eron, 1996; McCord, 1996) and engaging in criminal behavior as adults (Straus & Donnelly, 2001; Straus & Lauer, 1992).

You can say something like:

> "Children who get beaten (or spanked) at home are more likely to commit crimes as adults than children who experience attentive parenting *without* corporal punishment. I know you want your children to lead an upright life and stay out of trouble. There are other ways to help them do this."

## Improving Family Communication

Most parents would like to know about their children's concerns as they grow up. Parents who use corporal punishment on their young children may not consider the implications of this strategy as the children grow into their teens:

> "Your children are more likely to confide in you if they do not feel threatened by you. When they are teenagers and face difficult choices, they will not tell you what worries them if they are afraid of you."

Cultural minority parents often show great family loyalty and may be hesitant to criticize or even question the way they themselves were disciplined as children. Asking parents about what they felt and thought when they were punished physically as children facilitates exploration of relevant issues. They are apt to report *fear and anger*, although they may minimize these by saying that now they appreciate the way their parents taught them respect and the *difference between right and wrong*. We can suggest that it is possible to teach these important lessons without instilling fear, and that doing so will improve family communication and reduce estrangement and the possibility of negative psychological outcomes.

I sometimes ask parents, "Do you want your children to speak with you as they grow up about their concerns on important issues such as drugs, sex, relationships, and other conflicts they may be having?" Almost all parents agree that they do. Then I ask, "How can you keep a strong and open relationship with your children so they can approach you without fear around difficult issues? How can you communicate with them now so they won't want to lie to you when they're older?" When they hear the issue phrased in this way, many parents are able to see that the immediate goal of resolving a particular disciplinary incident needs to be viewed in the context of the longer term goal of maintaining an open and trusting relationship.

## Thinking of the Future

It can be hard for parents to envision their own children in the future as parents and part of a couple themselves. However, helping the parents consider the possible impact of their actions across the generations may move them to reconsider their use of physical force:

> "What would it be like if you could roll time forward, and discovered that your son was beating up his wife, and said that he learned to beat the people he loved at home from your example? Boys who are beaten are more likely to use violence with their wives when they grow up. And girls who are beaten are more likely to be victimized again as adults. Girls and boys who are beaten at home are more likely to beat their own children when they are parents."

Helping parents see the potential implications of their actions on future generations gives them pause to reconsider. And within that pause, change can happen.

## SUPPORTING NONVIOLENT PARENTING

The above ideas describe several ways that core values can be used to build parental opposition to corporal punishment. They are meant to be suggestive rather than exhaustive. I have heard Latino and African American parents comment that "White parents train their dogs but let their children run wild." Vietnamese parents also believe in children's obedience, citing the traditional saying, "Children sit where their parents place them." With families who value obedience, professionals need to emphasize that they too believe it is important for children to be given clear limits and know the difference between right and wrong (see Chapter 8, section on parenting groups). Some parents will welcome ideas about how to educate a child without corporal punishment. We can provide access to culturally sensitive parenting programs (e.g., Popkin, 1998), books (e.g., Faber & Mazlich, 1991), and examples of attentive parenting in popular culture (e.g., the televised *Cosby Show*).

For parents to give up corporal punishment, they need to establish an effective alternative system of instruction and discipline. Four different kinds of parenting behaviors contribute to such a system (Howard, 1996): those that promote the parent–child relationship (e.g., positive time together), those that avoid conflict (e.g., making sure the child is well rested and well fed), those that reinforce positive behaviors (e.g., praise, enjoyable time together), and those that decrease undesired behaviors (e.g., disincentives or punishments). Parents who resort to frequent or severe corporal punishment are likely to rely too much on punitive techniques at the expense of the other three avenues for influencing a child's behavior. Professionals who engage in parent education need to make sure they are not simply substituting one form of punishment (e.g., time-out) for another. Parents need to learn to engage in a broad range of responsive behaviors, of which punishment forms the smallest part.

Parents who agree to attempt to raise their children without corporal punishment deserve our support and empathy, especially during the transition period. A child's established negative behaviors often resist change, and may even initially worsen, causing parents to doubt the usefulness of abandoning corporal punishment. We need to help parents figure out ways to face these initial pressures and prevent the emergence of a new set of problems. Depending on the children's age, it can be helpful for parents to sit down with their children and explain that they will be trying something new, and why they want to change. They should try to enlist the children's understanding, support, and—eventually—forgiveness.

Parents may be subject to criticism and even scorn from their friends and family when they foreswear corporal punishment. Raising children is a community activity for many cultural minority families, where extended family members, friends, and even neighbors contribute to a child's upbringing through sharing resources and freely "correcting" unwanted behavior. A Puerto Rican who was raised in a small town on the Island said, "When I was a boy, I really had to stay out of trouble on my street because if I did anything wrong—whack! I could get it from any of my neighbors as easily as my parents. There was no hiding" (Roberto Irizarry, personal communication, April 1999). Some immigrants maintain this sense of a village for raising their children by living in tight-knit ethnic neighborhoods in the United States and Canada, where extended family members, godparents, and friends from the preimmigration community live within a few blocks of each other.

African American families, immigrants, and families from religious minority groups that rely heavily on corporal punishment may experience a sense of disorientation and outsider status as they begin to change their discipline norms. Over time the Johnson family, discussed at the beginning of this chapter, decided to stop using corporal punishment. They said they just became less comfortable with it. The mother confided in me, "I think we need a new group of friends who share our new values. It's too exhausting to explain to everybody all the time why we don't smack the kids. They accuse us of 'acting White.' I'm sick of it."

When discussing the sensitive topic of physical abuse, it is important to acknowledge the many strengths parents like the Johnsons may demonstrate, including physical affection, respect, generosity, paternal involvement, and close family ties. Most parents who use corporal punishment already shape their children's behavior in other ways (e.g., through praise and modeling). We should observe the *effective* ways parents teach and demonstrate affection toward their children, clearly point these out to parents, and encourage them to engage in these behaviors more deliberately and frequently. Also, we can show parents ways to vary and enhance existing skills by incorporating new skills. By taking this approach, we can avoid insulting parents' existing strategies, or recommending what they might perceive as impractical techniques. Finally, we may ask parents about their ideal for family functioning, and help them work through some of the stressors that may have pushed them to stray from their own ideal model. These stressors may include migration, job loss, a death, a separation or divorce—all of which could impel a family away from its own ideals.

## PREVENTION PROGRAMMING

Professionals should institute prevention programs designed to reach all parents (primarily prevention), as well as those parents considered to be at risk for physical abuse (secondary or targeted prevention) (see Chapter 8). Depending on their settings, professionals can offer parent education, social events, and community-building activities that decrease parental isolation and give parents an opportunity to learn about positive parenting. Some of these programs should be offered in languages other than English and directed to the specific needs of the immigrant population. For example, a school professional could offer a session on changing unwanted behaviors, or effective discipline with teenagers, or keeping the conversation going with your child. If these sessions are offered in a nonpathologizing way, with a correspondingly unoffensive name, parents are more likely to participate. For these efforts to succeed with members of cultural minority groups, we should enlist concerned parents from diverse groups to help plan the sessions and solicit participation personally among their neighbors and friends. The most effective teaching technique may be the affirmation by other parents from the same group that learning nonphysical forms of discipline is important and that these techniques do work.

The following case example illustrates many of the techniques described earlier, as well as some of the social stressors described below:

Cristina and her parents moved from Mexico to the United States when she was 14. Two years later, she spoke fluent English, demanded a telephone in her room, and acted like her peers born in the United States. In contrast, her parents, who were working in food service with other Latinos, spoke almost no English and found themselves increasingly dependent on Cristina's help as a linguistic and cultural interpreter. For example, only Cristina answered the telephone. If she wasn't home, her parents would just let it ring. Perhaps because she was an only child, Cristina's parents had raised her indulgently, rarely disciplining her physically and often working overtime to buy her clothes and shoes that were beyond their means. One day Cristina spoke in a way that her mother found disrespectful and ungrateful. Furious, her mother slapped her across the face, hard.

The next day at school Cristina showed her mark to her guidance counselor. The counselor called a meeting for after school that very day. The mother arrived at the counselor's office with a cousin—the father refused to attend. The mother said she wanted the cousin to interpret and asked the school's Spanish teacher, who was present to serve as an interpreter, to leave the room because she was afraid of gossip. The session lasted over an hour. Cristina and her mother wept profusely, moving quickly from blame about the specific incident to discussing their anguish about how their roles had changed since their move, and how difficult the parents' dependence on their daughter was becoming for all involved. The counselor listened empathically and helped the mother and daughter articulate how much they loved each other, but how much stress each was experiencing. They brainstormed ways to relieve Cristina of her parentified role. The counselor informed the family about a local social service agency for immigrants that provided many services, including interpreting and free classes in English as a second language.

Toward the middle of the hour, the counselor informed the mother that in the United States slapping a child hard across the face might be considered abusive. She affirmed the mother's loving parenting and the circumstances that led up to the slap. She informed the mother that she would have to call a state agency charged with protecting children. She placed the call while Cristina, her mother, and the cousin listened. At the end of the call, she reported to the family that the agency probably would not investigate this time, but that it would keep the family's name on file, to reconsider if there were further incidents. The counselor told Cristina that she did the right thing in seeking help, and the mother agreed. Although there were further conflicts between the daughter and her parents, as can be expected in any family, the parents never resorted to violence again.

In the above example, we see a family that has strayed from its own ideal form of parenting, partly because of immigration stress. The counselor helped the family identify its stressors and experience emotional closeness. The counselor explained the workings of the child protection system in the United States, fulfilled her legal obligation, referred the family to appropriate resources, and established a warm personal relationship with the family members who were present. All this was accomplished in one extended family session, followed by brief contacts with the daughter throughout the school year.

## CONCLUDING THOUGHTS

This chapter is necessarily only a partial examination of all the factors contributing to decisions about corporal punishment and physical abuse, decisions that must be made by cultural minority families and professionals alike. For example, this chapter fails to address the challenges of working in families where wife-battering and physical child abuse occur together, which is the case in approximately half of all child-abusing families (Shipman, Rossman, & West, 1999). Essentially, as long as there is violence in the couple, efforts to end physical child abuse are likely to be ineffective. The battered woman will be afraid to challenge her partner, and may inflict abuse on her children herself. Also, this chapter does not cover situations where physical and sexual child abuse co-occur, necessitating a more comprehensive and extensive intervention.

In sum, I recommend that professionals do the following when concerned about the harshness or frequency of physical discipline in a cultural minority family:

1. Join with all members of the family by interacting with them in a warm, professional manner. Remember that the relationships established with *all* members of the family are of utmost importance.

2. Ask in a nonblaming way about the incident or incidents that raised concern (following state guidelines pertaining to reporting child abuse and neglect). If it is necessary to file a report, you should do so in the most supportive way possible.

3. Briefly assess the parents, the child, their relationships, and the major stressors in the family's life (Fontes, 2000). If the people and relationships are essentially stable and loving, follow the steps below (a, b, c). If the family evidences severe psychological disturbance, other forms of violence, substance abuse, or unmanageable chaos, more comprehensive interventions and referrals may be required.

   a. Discuss with the parents the ways their current disciplinary practices are and are not working for them. Suggest that effective alternatives will better prepare the child for future success and achievement, and will protect the family from further government intervention.

   b. Engage with the parents in using alternatives to corporal punishment and monitoring their success. Help parents notice and celebrate each small move toward parenting without violence.

   c. Help the parents reduce their isolation and stress.

When offered with an attitude of genuine caring, these interventions should enable you to help members of ethnic and religious minority groups raise their children without violence.

## QUESTIONS TO THINK ABOUT AND DISCUSS

1. What kinds of punishment were used in your family or your ethnic group when you were a child?

2. Remember and describe a time when you were punished physically as a child (or when you witnessed a child being punished physically). What happened and how did it make you feel at the time?

3. How do your own personal experiences of corporal punishment affect your professional work on this issue? Do these experiences make it harder or easier to work with people from specific cultural groups?

4. How would you work with a family that insists on its legal right to use corporal punishment, but has been physically abusive on at least one occasion?

5. Describe the relationship between corporal punishment and physical abuse.

6. Do you agree or disagree with the following statement, and why: "Children should never be spanked or slapped for purposes of education or control."

# CHAPTER SIX

# Child Sexual Abuse

In this chapter I discuss some of the issues that arise when working with people from cultural minority groups on issues of child sexual abuse. I have chosen the concept of shame as a way to organize the material, recognizing that entire books have been written about culturally competent approaches to child sexual abuse intervention (Fontes, 1995a; Lewis, 1999). In this chapter I discuss ways professionals can work productively with diverse clients to overcome the harmful effects of child sexual abuse. (While most of the examples in this chapter concern the sexual abuse of girls by boys and men, because this is the most common situation, other examples are also included, particularly in the section on predictions of a shameful future.) I have chosen to focus on shame because of its centrality as an emotion in sexual abuse, because of the importance of addressing it in treatment with victims and survivors, and because of the ways cultural minority status can intensify shame, as I hope becomes clear below.

Definitions of shame vary, but they share the notion that the shamed person's core being has been maligned. Holzman (1995) describes shame in the following way:

> The focus is not on the harm done to others, but on the defect in myself. Shame involves feelings of exposure and an impulse to hide. . . . Irrational shame is a feeling of having been exposed as a fundamentally and irremediably defective human being. (p. 326)

Shame and honor are seen as being opposites, with honor as the highest goal consisting of "a claim to worth along with the social acknowledgment of worth" (Emory University, 1999). In contrast, shame is the feeling of no claim to worth, exacerbated by the lack of social acknowledgment of worth. That is, not only does a shamed person feel unworthy inside him- or herself, the person also feels he or she lacks worth in others' eyes.

When working with someone who has been hurt by child sexual abuse, it is important to ask, "What was most difficult about this experience for you?" Such a question helps us move from thinking that we know about child sexual abuse generally to knowing about this particular person's experience in all of its personal and cultural individuality.

For one child victim of incest, the "most difficult" thing will be adjusting to a new teacher if the father is forced to leave the household, the family moves in with relatives, and the child has to change schools. For another, it will be the nightmares. For a third, it might be that her mother will not allow her to play with her cousins as punishment for disclosing and breaking up the family. For a fourth, it might be the teasing he is subjected to, as everyone in the neighborhood calls him a "faggot" because he was abused by a man.

As children suffer in distinct ways, so do adults and families. For one adult survivor, the worst part will be fear that this experience has permanently and irrevocably impaired her sexual functioning or made her unlovable. For another, it will be the continued strained relations she experiences with family members who were either involved in the abuse or who failed to protect her. For one family whose child has been victimized, the worst part will be acknowledging that they have failed to protect their child. For another family, it will be their inability to protect themselves from intrusive and shaming interactions with the child welfare system.

Clearly, our efforts to help people affected by sexual abuse should begin with making sure the child is safe. Then we should continue on to the aspects of the situation that are identified as most problematic by the people involved. People of all cultural backgrounds are more likely to benefit from and cooperate with services if these services are directed toward meeting their own priorities.

While the concerns of people affected by sexual abuse vary widely, common themes do recur. Many excellent sources provide information on individual (Friedrich, 1995b; Gil, 1996b), family (Gil, 1996a; Trepper & Barrett, 1989), and group (Friedrich, 1990) intervention for sexual child abuse. This chapter cannot begin to convey or even outline these approaches. Rather, in this chapter I address some of the relevant cultural issues around *shame*—a core issue that is common to many child victims, adult survivors, their families, and others affected by sexual abuse, and an issue that has been found to be key in adjustment following sexual abuse.

## SHAME IN CHILD SEXUAL ABUSE

In a study of 147 child and adolescent victims who were assessed upon discovery of sexual abuse and 1 year later, degree of shame and attributional style were found to be the greatest determinants of adjustment (Feiring, Taska, & Lewis, 2002).[1] Those children who exhibited a reduction in shame a year after the abuse showed improved adjustment. The degree of shame and attributional style were found to be even more important than the severity of the abuse in determining how children fared.

By their very nature, interactions related to child sexual abuse are rife with shame for most people touched by it. Victims feel ashamed because they have participated in taboo activities, and often have maintained secrecy about those activities. For example, a stepfather may perform fellatio on his 8-year-old stepson, and then tell the boy to keep it a secret from his mother. So the boy becomes ashamed of having been involved in a taboo act (sex with another male), for having violated a social boundary (sex with his stepfather), and also for having betrayed his relationship with his mother by keeping a secret from her and by being involved with *her* sexual partner. The boy's shame is apt to further isolate him from his mother and from other potential sources of support. I am reminded of a young Mexican boy who—in giving a statement after repeated sexual abuse by his stepfather—said, "And I'm not gay or anything." Because this victim had participated in an activity considered "bad" and deviant in his culture, he considered himself "bad" and deviant—by thinking that the activity was a reflection on *his* sexual self, rather than that of the offender.

Victims are shamed by statements made by the offender, who will often try to convince victims that they provoked the abuse and are responsible for it. For instance, an offender might say, "You know you're asking for it, wearing those tight little shorts." Such a statement leads a victim to believe that—indeed—she did in some away bring about the abuse. She may try to ward off future assaults by changing the way she dresses, only to have the offender find another way to pin responsibility on her during the next encounter ("You know you were asking for it, the way you looked at me"). If she believes that she was responsible for the abuse, then she can believe that she has some possible control over future assaults—if only she could find the right way out. The offender may also perform particularly degrading acts with the victim or reward her financially for her participation, both of which increase her feelings of shame.

The responses of those who discover the abuse can also shame a victim. A nonoffending mother will often yell at a child for not having spoken up sooner, or for having "been willing to" go along with the offender's requests. Nonoffending family members are ashamed of not having been able to protect their children and of having stains on their sense of family normalcy. The easiest and most accessible target for their anger is often the victimized child.

---

[1] *Attributions* refers to the child's explanation of why the abuse occurred.

Behind the various points I make in this book are a plea and a set of ideas for moving from shame-based to empowerment-based encounters around child abuse with immigrant and cultural minority families. A simple visit by a law enforcement officer or a child protection worker is an occasion for shame for most families. Since only "bad" parents would be questioned by these authorities, then the very inquiry by authorities can feel like a shameful accusation of parental inadequacy.

This situation may feel particularly painful for those clients who come from cultures that are highly organized around honor and shame, such as most Asian cultures and many Muslim and Latin American cultures. Sitting in the waiting room of an agency geared to the investigation or treatment of child abuse is embarrassing and shameful for many families, as they hope ardently that no one they know will see them there. Also, the simple mentioning of the body parts involved in the incident will be shaming to many victims, who may have been taught that discussing these parts and these acts is a disgrace—a fall from grace (see Chapter 4).

The shame around child sexual abuse seems almost contagious. Professionals who work in this area may share it by refusing to speak publicly about their own experiences of abuse. Police officers, psychologists, social workers, and others who work in this area sometimes say that child sexual abuse is considered one of the least prestigious areas of professional concern. Learning to interview children well just does not carry the same cachet at the police academy as learning to "break down" suspects in an interrogation.

As professionals, we are accustomed to asking people about the most personal of matters—for example, relationships, money, sex, violence, and hygiene—and it is easy for us to forget how intimate these topics really are and how invasive our questions may feel. We collect the most private details into a file or "case," which we then tuck away in a drawer or present to our colleagues, impersonally. If we were to look hard at the cases in our file drawers that contains details of some of the most horrific kinds of pain imaginable, we could not help but experience awe. As we ask question after question, gathering information, our clients feel us probing into a deep and secret place, even if we sometimes forget the emotional impact of our discussion. In her novel *Push* (1996), about the recovery from incest of an illiterate teenage African American girl, Sapphire writes in the girl's voice about the disempowerment and shame she feels in being asked questions before admittance into an educational program:

> I wonder what exactly do file say. I know it say I got a baby. Do it say who Daddy? What kinda baby? Do it say how pages the same for me, how much I weigh, fights I done had? I don't know what file say. I do know every time they wants to fuck wif me or decide something in my life, here they come wif the

mutherfucking file. Well, OK, they got file, know every mutherfucking thing. (p. 28)

We must proceed with the utmost care as we ask questions, acknowledging the private and taboo nature of many of the topics we are exploring. We must ask in ways that are as uninvasive and unintrusive as possible. We must allow our clients to recount and evaluate their experiences at their own pace. Our questions must affirm the worth and value of the people to whom they are posed, rather than shaming them.

## CULTURAL ASPECTS OF SHAME IN CHILD SEXUAL ABUSE

The shame around sexual abuse intersects with ethnic culture in many ways. Here I address responsibility for the abuse, failure to protect, fate, damaged goods, virginity, predictions of a shameful future, revictimization, and the layers of shame produced by cultural oppression—with an eye on how these affect members of cultural minority groups who have been impacted by sexual abuse.

Some of the components of shame—like the sense of being permanently damaged—are common to most victims of sexual child abuse regardless of their cultural or ethnic background. But the way people experience that feeling of being damaged, and the way it is handled by others, varies with ethnic culture. There are also cultural elements—such as a cultural emphasis on the importance of virginity—and systemic elements—such as discrimination by social services, schools, and the police—that can intensify the shame felt by cultural minority victims of child sex abuse and their families. Learning how to ease the shame is one of the keys for professionals to help struggling victims recover.

### Responsibility for the Abuse

When a child has been abused sexually, all parties involved look for someone to blame. Frequently, offenders accuse their victims of being flirtatious or seductive or "asking for it." Most children seek affection. If they receive sexual abuse instead, they may come to believe it was their desire for closeness that brought about the sexual acts. Children become confused and ashamed about the sexual incidents. In an effort to feel that they have some control over the incidents, they may develop the belief that they brought them about. If they experienced bodily pleasure or accepted gifts or participated in multiple episodes, they may feel especially ashamed. This is particularly hard for children when—as is usually the case—the offender does not take responsibility for his acts and—as is often the case—the nonffending parent and others who learn of the abuse are not clear in placing responsibility squarely on the shoulders of the person who has offended.

The assignment of responsibility for the abuse can vary widely across cultures. In many traditional cultures, sexual relations are viewed as a fundamental struggle: something females should try to avoid and males of all ages should try to obtain. The value of a boy or man's masculinity may hinge on the number of his conquests, and the value of a girl or woman's femininity may hinge on her chastity. (Some would argue that these same values hold true in U.S. and Canadian secondary schools where boys gain prestige if they are considered "players" and girls lose prestige if they are considered "sluts.") Where sexual acts have occurred outside marriage, the girl or woman is assumed to have made herself accessible and is often held responsible, even when there is a difference in age or power between the people involved. The belief that they are responsible for the abuse can lead victimized girls to feel great shame. One Puerto Rican social worker described the sexual education of children in traditional Latino families in this way:

> "And they teach their children to have the most traditional attitudes; they educate them to be enemies. The girls have to keep their legs closed, because the boys are raised so that if the girls open them, they're going to take advantage of it. And that's the sexual education that they get. It's not that there is no sexual education, it's that what they get is bad. The education that they get is that if you expose yourself you're going to suffer because [the boys] cannot control themselves. And besides, the boys have permission to do what they want."

A Peruvian woman told me about how her brother had been found to be having sexual relations with his 9-year-old stepdaughter, and how the girl was then banished to a convent. "It wasn't his fault!," she insisted. "The girl was right there with him and was very pretty. She wore short dresses. She sat on his lap. She asked him to tuck her in at night. Her mother was away for a month. He couldn't help himself!" In the abstract, I expect this woman would have asserted that a man who engaged in sexual relations with a child was responsible for this act. But because the offense was committed by her brother, whom she loved, she assigned the girl the role of temptress and was therefore able to maintain her closeness to her brother.

Even a young girl who has been sexually abused or raped may be held at least partly responsible for what happened, but I believe this attitude is even more prevalent when the victim shows signs of physical maturation.

She may be told, "Nothing enters where it isn't invited." This attitude increases her shame and the likelihood that she will keep silent about what has happened to her. If girls are taught that they are responsible for guarding their sexuality from older men including their fathers, and that men cannot control their desire when faced with anything that looks like a provocation by a girl, it is a small leap for girls to blame themselves when abuse does occur.

According to a Colombian social worker, some mothers of victims—many of whom were victimized themselves—covertly or overtly blame their children for the sexual acts that have occurred:

> "I still see women in the clinic saying, 'And I told her that she shouldn't go out like that! That she shouldn't open the door, or that she should lock the door to sleep! I have been telling her that for ages ever since she was a little girl!'"

The idea that the child rather than the adult is responsible for sexual acts between them is a common myth that serves to protect adults from their own feelings of shame for having failed to protect a vulnerable child. An important part of recovery for many survivors is to learn and truly come to believe that they were not responsible for the abuse. When responsibility and blame can be properly assigned to the offenders, victims are able to release some of the shame that binds them.

It is important for professionals to understand cultural norms around the assignation of blame and responsibility. At the same time, professionals need to help their clients place responsibility for past incidents squarely on the shoulders of the person who has offended, and make a number of different family members take responsibility for future protection of the child.

Whether working with adult survivors, child victims, or their families, many professionals choose to use a deliberate, concrete strategy to help clients reassign responsibility appropriately. For instance, a therapist might help a child draw a picture of the offender and the child standing next to each other (stick figures are fine). The therapist leads the child to indicate the height differential between the two. Then the child is asked to indicate the weights, the ages, and any other aspects of the two that illustrate their power differences.

Depending on the child's age, the therapist asks a series of questions that help the child understand the power differential, such as, "Who can lift something heavier? Who knows more words? Who is old enough to hold a job? Who has been to more places? Who is a grownup? Whose job is it to make sure children are safe? Who is old enough to vote and make other big decisions?" These strategies can help victims discard irrational beliefs that they themselves were responsible for the abuse. A therapist can direct a similar series of questions to a nonoffending parent who blames the victim. For instance, "If your daughter and your husband had set the house on fire while they were playing with matches, who would you think is responsible?" Or, "If your son wanted to drive and your boyfriend handed him the keys to the car, and he got into an accident, who would be responsible?"

It may be particularly difficult for families to assign blame appropriately in cases of brother–sister incest, particularly in cultures that value boys more highly than girls. Although research reveals few differences between brother–sister incest and father–daughter incest in terms of its traumatic impact (Cyr, Wright, McDuff, & Perron, 2002), parents frequently minimize or deny the significance of brother–sister incest, or they blame the girl. It may be helpful to underscore the point that boys who molest their sisters may go on to molest others, and that it is in the boy's as well as the girl's best interests to address the molestation directly rather than to pretend it did not occur.

## Failure to Protect

Nonoffending family members are often ashamed of having failed to protect a child from sexual abuse—thereby having proved themselves inadequate in a key task of their cultural roles as mothers, fathers, older brothers, and so on. For instance, ideas of machismo—common in many Latino, Arab, and other cultures—dictate that men are responsible for protecting their wives and families (De Young & Zigler, 1994). A man whose child has been victimized may feel like a failure as a man; his sense of failure could easily drive him to suicide, or to physically attacking the sexual offender to recover his feelings of dignity and self-worth. One Latino man said that if he found out his child had been abused sexually, he'd lose his mind and "black out" (Fontes, Cruz, & Tabachnik, 2001). Another said he'd gladly spend his life in jail for killing a sexual offender. A third said, "I would report. But frankly, if it was with a child in my family, I would kill. I'd put a stick up his ass to see how he feels—what he's done." Some African American men responded similarly when confronted with the same scenario. One said, "You got so much anger in you, you can't even think about calling no agency." Others described being able to put brakes on their actions:

> "Human nature would make me really angry. But I'd have to really sit down and pray and allow God to give me peace of mind so I can look at the situation as a whole: my kid or someone else's kid."

While anger against the perpetrator is natural, and feelings of inadequacy related to failure to protect are understandable, men must be made to see that retaliating physically and becoming further entangled in the legal and criminal justice system is apt to increase—rather than decrease—the child victim's distress. Professionals need to show fathers and other concerned adults ways in which they can actively and positively participate in the child victim's recovery and protect other children (Pearce & Pezzot-Pearce, 1997). When working with nonoffending men from cultures with a tradition of machismo, it may be especially important to help them find active ways to assert their power for future protection and recovery, rather than resorting to vengeance.

## Fate

The dominant U.S. and Canadian cultures emphasize individual control and responsibility, as illustrated in the Horatio Alger myth of an individual achieving success through hard work and the general glorification of myths of Lone Ranger individuals who make it on their own, without help from others or God. In contrast, other cultures have an external locus of control, believing that forces outside or beyond an individual determine the life course. Sue and Sue (2003) describe the different forms this external locus of control can take, including chance and luck (the idea that one's future is controlled by chance occurrences), benevolent cultural dictates (such as God's will), or political forces (such as a realistic appraisal of the limitations that discrimination and poverty impose). Misunderstandings can result when a professional with an internal locus of control and responsibility (who believes that one is the master of one's own fate and is solely responsible for one's situation) works with a client with an external locus of control and responsibility (who may see limitations on one's power over one's destiny).

Many Latinos will add "*Si Diós quiere*" (If God is willing) to any statement regarding the future, such as, "I'll see you tomorrow, God willing." Arabic speakers will add a similar phrase, "*Inshallah*." People with this culturally fatalistic view will often respond quite passively in the face of a discovery of sexual abuse. This passivity could be a culturally induced fatalism, or could stem from confusion and shock about the accusations, fear of authorities, and other factors discussed in Chapter 2. (Even when cultures seem to hold a fatalistic worldview, there usually are also cultural elements admonishing people to take responsibility for their lives. For instance, Muslims are traditionally admonished, "Don't leave your camel untied." That is, people must take responsibility for their own lives, even as they respect Allah's power.)

Southeast Asian parents may respond with a striking lack of apparent sympathy to a child victim of sexual abuse, believing that this misfortune surely results from karma—it must be a punishment on the child and/or family for wrongdoings committed in a previous incarnation. If knowledge of the sexual abuse were to become public in their ethnic community, the family might be ostracized and considered unworthy, because of this karmic stain. The girl would also lose part of her potential value as a future daughter-in-law—an important part of a grown woman's identity. Viewed in this light, there is a lot of stigma attached to misfortunes such as sexual abuse or having a disability.

I have heard child protection workers describe Cambodian parents as uncaring because they did not seem to object to the worker's removal of the child from the home, and they neither challenged nor complied with the instructions about how to regain custody. In this case, the parents had already had their families yanked apart during the brutal rule of the Khmer Rouge in Cambodia (Scully, Kuoch, & Miller, 1995). They had been threatened and beaten by gun-wielding authorities in Cambodia and in Thai refugee camps, and had been at the mercy of authorities upon entry into the United States. The strategy they had learned—one that had served them well in these other situations—was silent compliance. They had learned to view circumstances as beyond their control. Their passive acquiescence was misinterpreted by U.S. professionals as lack of caring.

Catholics frequently assume that sexual abuse is either God's will or a test from God. A Guatemalan mother may throw up her hands and say, "This is what God wants," or "This is my cross to bear." Family members often believe that the abuse is God's message to them, and have trouble placing their children's concerns at the center of the story. For example, a mother may believe that her daughter's sexual abuse is divine retribution for an indiscretion that she herself had committed, or a father might believe that God is punishing him for something he did by making his own child into a victim. One Catholic Mexican mother explained her husband's sexual abuse of their daughter as God's way of telling the father to stop drinking so much (De La Cruz-Quiroz, 2000). These attributions of responsibility to God may be seen as an attempt to make meaning of an incomprehensible event.

How should we handle these attributions of responsibility? First, we must become aware of them. We should inquire of each person involved in the intervention, "How do you explain why the abuse happened?"

Then, if we learn that a client is attributing the abuse to God, destiny, karma, or something else over which he may believe he has little future control, a "both/and" approach might be helpful. In this approach we acknowledge the client's attributions, and at the same time help him reach other conclusions about it as well. For instance, we can listen respectfully to the client's explanation for the occurrence, and acknowledge its importance. Then we can follow it up with a statement like this:

> "Thank you for letting me know how you explain what happened. I'd like to suggest a couple of other ideas, so you can know how I think about it. I expect that both perspectives contain some truth. _____ chose to abuse your child because _____ has sexual feelings toward children, and found a way to be alone with your child and act on those feelings. We can work together to help your child and family recover from this, and to make sure nothing like this happens again. I encourage you to continue to do all the things you are doing that are helping you cope [e.g., praying]. I have ideas about other things that could be helpful to you and your child too, and have been helpful to other people in your situation."

We are unlikely to be able to change a family member or victim's entire worldview, and this probably would not be desirable anyway. Rather, clients can be encouraged to rely both on traditional beliefs and sources of support and also on child abuse professionals (Taylor & Fontes, 1995). "If we are physically ill, first we pray, then we find the best physician available. If our cars are emitting black smoke, we pray and find a good mechanic" (p. 188). Similarly, adults faced with the sexual abuse of their loved ones can both accept their fate and work to improve their children's future. Clients should not be shamed for their culturally learned response to the abuse. Rather, they can be invited into additional ways of looking at the abuse that might help their children's recovery.

## Damaged Goods

A 22-year-old female Puerto Rican victim of sexual abuse told me: "When something like this happens to you, you don't just lose your virginity, you lose so much! You lose your rights! And you are like a zombie: you're living but you're not."

This sense of being soiled or spoiled often starts with the first sexual assault. "I felt bad. Each time he touched me, I felt like what I wanted was to bathe, to wash, to clean myself," said one Puerto Rican adult survivor. When the abuse occurs repeatedly, often over a period of years, the sense of being defiled seems to rub into the very fiber of victims so they no longer think of themselves as having been dirtied, but rather define their very being as dirty. This ashamed feeling seems global and unchanging—they feel that they are wholly unworthy and always will be. For decades after the abuse has stopped, they may continue to view themselves as ruined.

Psychotherapists who hope to help victims overcome this feeling of being dirtied as a result of the abuse may need to spend some time focusing on the sexual aspect of the abuse. Victims who had orgasms, who solicited the abuse at particular times, or who complied with it over a period of time are likely to feel particularly ashamed. The resolution to these feelings of being dirty may include a cultural element. For instance, a Jewish person who has been sexually abused may wish to mark her freedom from shame by immersing in the *mikvah,* or traditional bath (this would, of course, follow exploration of the topic in treatment). Similarly, receiving communion may be particularly significant to a Catholic victim who—for a time—felt that his or her participation in the abuse was a sin. Psychotherapists may ask their clients if they think there are aspects of their culture or religion which can help the clients feel complete, whole, and clean again, and then co-construct meaningful rituals or ceremonies with their clients incorporating these elements.

## Virginity

Most sexual abuse of children does not involve penetration. However, the specter of loss of virginity for girls assumes great importance, regardless.

Many cultures control women's sexuality by expecting girls to maintain their virginity until marriage. This expectation spans the oceans and includes traditional families from many parts of Asia, Africa, Europe, the Middle East, and the Americas. Virginity is also being revived as a cultural value among some groups in the United States. "Abstinence only" curricula are frequently replacing comprehensive sexuality education in U.S. schools, and teenagers are encouraged to take "pledges of virginity." (The proponents of these approaches have failed to consider their potential impact on children in the classroom who have been sexually abused and are receiving the message that they are less valuable than their nonassaulted, virgin peers.)[2]

In some traditional cultures, a girl who has engaged in any kind of sexual activity—even against her will—may be perceived as losing her virginity, and thereby be considered either not suitable for marriage or of lesser value as a bride. Christian girls from various denominations are frequently advised to pray for forgiveness for the sin of their abuse. In some cultures, such as parts of Sudan, Iran, Saudi Arabia, Pakistan, and Nigeria, where the Sharia form of Islam is practiced, a girl who is abused sexually

---

[2]In her study of parenting teens, McDonald (2004) found that most of the teens first received sex education in school *after* they had been sexually abused. The notion of abstinence—which implies that the teens should resist a temptation—simply did not seem to apply to their circumstances. Most of the teens became pregnant or were sexually abused by men who were quite a bit older, and in circumstances that included coercion. They were not giving in to temptation; rather, they were giving in to fear, violence, or the need to escape from an intolerable home situation.

may be considered guilty of sex outside marriage, and therefore subject to being lashed publicly or stoned to death. Yuksel (2000) describes the importance of virginity among the majority Muslim population in Turkey:

> In many places the absence of virginity may mean that a young girl loses her chance for marriage. If the situation is known, she loses her prestige within the family [just] as the family loses it in their close neighborhood. . . . Sexual abusers seem to pay attention to this issue, and some girls are threatened with "losing their hymen" which explains [the elevated presence of] nonpenetrative sexual abuse. On the other hand, the first reaction of the nonoffending parent and other relatives is to take the child or young girl for an examination of her virginity, when they find out about the abuse. If the hymen is left intact, the sexual abuse cannot be proved, and this makes the denial easier for the family. Professionals, therefore, emphasize the fact that the presence of the hymen does not preclude sexual abuse. (p. 157)

Even in families that have rejected other aspects of traditional life, this emphasis on virginity can persist, as I saw myself when working on a psychiatric crisis team in New England years ago:

> One night I was called to a hospital to assess the 45-year-old daughter of Italian immigrants who had tried to kill herself by ingesting painkillers. She reported that her mother had just died, and she had no one else to love and never would. She eventually also reported that she had been raped by a family friend at the age of 8, and had never told anyone. She said she knew that she would never be able to get married because of the rape, and therefore had never pursued a romantic relationship. Instead, she had dedicated herself to her church and caring for her parents. Now that they were both gone, she saw no hope of further intimacy.

To this day, I remember this woman with great sorrow. The course of her life and all her relationships had been altered by an early sexual assault that she had confided to no one. The cultural and religious emphasis on virginity had led her to believe that she had sinned and was different from other girls who had not been sexually assaulted. Her deep shame and suffering could have been avoided with proper intervention.

In her novel about a young Haitian girl who moves to New York, Edwidge Danticat (1994) movingly describes how a mother feels compelled to follow a cultural tradition related to virginity. The mother explains to her daughter:

> When I was a girl, my mother used to test us to see if we were virgins. She would put her finger in our very private parts and see if it would go inside. Your Tante

> Atie hated it. She used to scream like a pig in a slaughterhouse. The way my mother was raised, a mother is supposed to do that to her daughter until the daughter is married. It is her responsibility to keep her pure. (pp. 60–61)

When at a later point the daughter finally fails this test, the mother kicks the daughter out of the house, leaving her vulnerable to sexual and other exploitation. This digital "test" of virginity is apt to be considered a form of sexual assault by the courts, and may be perceived as just another rationalization or justification by people who work with sexual offenders. However, it also reveals a cultural truth about the importance of the hymen as "evidence" of sexual purity. I have heard of similar tests being performed in various cultures throughout the world and in families from a variety of cultures in the United States and Canada.

A Puerto Rican woman who had been abused sexually by her father for years describes the importance of her "lost" virginity in her life in terms of her husband's view of her childhood sexual abuse:

> "Often I think that as a man he—unconsciously—couldn't accept me, and that's why he did the things he did to me: the physical abuse, the sexual abuse, the emotional abuse—that is, the constant abuse. . . . He, as a Puerto Rican man, could have a lot of little girlfriends and go to bed with a whole bunch of women, but when the time comes to get married, he wants a pure woman. And since I wasn't pure in his view, because—as is said in Puerto Rico—*no me rompió la chapita* [he didn't pop my cherry] that probably bothered him. . . . Often he would tell me that he wanted to get divorced because he wanted to marry a woman he had dishonored the year before."

The emphasis on virginity leads to negative predictions about the future for a girl who has disclosed sexual abuse. These comments confirm for her that not only is she damaged in her own eyes, but others see her that way too. One therapist described the situation of a 12-year-old Puerto Rican girl who became pregnant after a rape by a neighbor, and was forced to have an abortion: "All her life from then on they would tell her that she couldn't wear white to her wedding because she was no longer a virgin. . . . No one ever asked her or helped her or anything." The girl was considered spoiled for marriage.

Particularly for individuals with less education, virginity as symbolized by the intactness of the hymen assumes great importance. One mother of a sexually abused preschooler emerged smiling from her conversation with the medical specialist who had interviewed and examined her daughter. The assessment confirmed that the girl's stepfather had fondled her and forced her to view pornography on numerous occasions, but the mother clapped her hands with delight because the girl still was a "señorita"—her hymen was intact.

The emphasis on virginity can make it difficult for children to disclose ("My parents will kill me, or him, if they find out!") and can make it difficult for family members to press charges or cooperate with treatment. Family members may worry that cooperating with authorities will make it more likely that word will get out that their daughter has been ruined. In an article on sexual abuse in Arab families in Israel, Baker, and Dwairy (2003) write about how the marriage prospects of *all* siblings in a family may be ruined if word gets out that one of the daughters has been victimized—the entire family is considered tainted.

Among Latinas, the sexual nature of sexual assault is often extremely important. Traditionally, women are supposed to be virgins until they marry and to remain completely faithful to their husband afterward. Sexual contact with another man—even if it was forcible rape—may make her feel ashamed and dirty down to her core. She may believe God will punish her for the assault, or she may believe the assault is punishment for something she has done or failed to do—perhaps she did not say enough Hail Marys, or had entertained thoughts of a man other than her husband, or had neglected to send money home to her parents that month. Her sense of shame may be worse if she did not physically resist the assault. She may have been made to engage in sexual acts that she feels are sinful, such as anal or oral sex. She may not even have the words to describe what happened, and certainly may feel too ashamed to tell. Latinas are raised to avoid "talking dirty," and so she may hesitate to tell you the sexual details of what happened. These same details may cause her anguish.

## Working with Concerns about Virginity

If family members place great value on virginity, professionals cannot simply ignore or dismiss these concerns. Rather, we must find ways to incorporate discussion and perhaps redefinition of virginity into our work with victims and their families. One therapist worked at redefining virginity for a 13-year-old Latina client who had been sexually abused, shifting the definition of virginity away from the concrete physical level of the hymen to a more relational or spiritual level:

> "We started talking about virginity and what that meant. My message to her was that virginity is not in your hymen but that it's really in your mind, and that I really considered her to be a virgin because she had not voluntarily had sex. . . . It was that 'damaged goods' issue. She was in tears. I was almost in tears. Really, I can't convey in words what it was like, but it was like this realization that there was some-

thing defective in her. Somehow the sexual part of her was not as valuable as her friend's. 'I'm used already, so it really doesn't matter,' the girl said, to explain why she had become sexually promiscuous."

Medical personnel are sometimes puzzled by family members' insistence on knowing whether a girl is "intact" or whether there is physical evidence of penetration. Medical examinations can rarely determine this with certainty (Jenny, 2002). One physician who works frequently with Vietnamese and Mexican immigrants, two groups that may be highly concerned with this question, describes how she responds:

> "If there is clear evidence of vaginal penetration and the family wants to know, I will say that with my highly specialized instrument, I was able to detect some evidence of penetration. I let them know that without this special instrument, I would not have been able to tell. I add that these tissues are full of blood and highly pliable at this age and that they will recover. I tell them that she will be able to marry and conduct relations like anyone else, and that no one will be able to detect a difference. I encourage them *not* to discuss with others the details of her assault, other than to say that physically she is fine. This usually relieves their anxiety and helps them treat her more normally."

## Predictions of a Shameful Future: Promiscuity, Homosexuality, and Sexual Offending

People from many cultures believe that girls who have suffered sexual abuse are likely to become promiscuous and boys who have been sexually abused by men are likely to become either homosexuals or sexual offenders. It's as if they will become "hooked" on taboo sexual activities.

Irene, a Puerto Rican who disclosed at the age of 15 that she had been sexually abused by her father for 6 years, was given tranquilizers and birth control pills covertly by her mother for the next several years:

> "I spent all my time drugged up. So in the morning every morning before she went to work my mother told me, 'Take this vitamin to build strength.' I took birth control pills for many years without knowing what they were. I didn't even know that birth control pills existed!"

On the day of Irene's wedding, her mother told her that she had been giving her birth control pills on a daily basis for years. Irene described this knowledge as extremely painful.

> "It was like, 'Now she must be running with other men and I don't want her knocked up. So let's give her pills.' That was the feeling."

As a group, girls who have been sexually abused do tend to engage in earlier and higher-risk sexual behaviors than girls who were not sexually abused (see section below on revictimization). However, this outcome is not inevitable, and is entirely avoidable if girls are given nonshaming support to understand what has happened to them and their often-confusing feelings around the incidents, and guidance on nonrisky ways to explore their sexual and romantic feelings. When they are ashamed of their participation in the abuse, and ashamed about sexual feelings that may have been awakened during the abuse, they may be more likely to "act out" these feelings in ways that put them at risk. I am reminded of a Puerto Rican family with whom I worked where one of the daughters had been fondled by her mother's former boyfriend. The girl disclosed when her mother broke up with the man. The girl never received counseling for this abuse and was told to "forget it," just as the mother had "forgotten" her own experiences of childhood abuse. At 12, the girl again disclosed fondling by a family friend. By this time the girl had passed through puberty and the mother saw her as responsible for her own actions with the man. Three years later, when the girl was 15, the mother was appalled to discover that the girl was having consensual sex with her boyfriend. This was considered a source of shame: the girl's and the entire family's reputation and honor were at stake.

On the other hand, 15-year-old Samantha was fondled by a neighbor once when she was baby-sitting for the neighbor's child. She told her parents the next day, and they reported the incident to the police. Samantha participated in a number of counseling sessions related to the abuse, and reports that she does not believe it has affected her in any way over the long term. Samantha was from a family that trusted the police and saw their daughter as having been victimized rather than corrupted. This attitude helped her recover.

Families from traditional cultures may view grimly any sign of sexual activity or interest in unmarried girls. They may punish two children who are caught with their pants down, so to speak, rather than inquiring as to whether the participation was mutual or coerced, and whether one child was victimized during the interaction.

Immigrant families often severely punish the sexual play or acting out that may follow abuse. The prohibitions against masturbating, particularly for girls, may run deep. In her novel *Dreaming in Cuban* (1992), Cristina García writes about the protagonist's mother finding her diary, where she had confessed that she enjoyed positioning herself just right in the shower, to feel pleasure between her legs:

> Now, whenever I'm in the bathroom, my mother knocks on the door like President Nixon's here and needs to use the john. . . . When Mom first found out about me in the tub, she beat me in the face and pulled my hair out in big

clumps. She called me a *desgraciada* and ground her knuckles into my temples. Then she forced me to work in her bakery every day after school. (p. 27)

Traditional parents may need guidance to understand the most helpful responses to normal sexual behavior in children (Johnson, 1999). They may also need some detailed suggestions as to how to respond to the sexualized behavior that sometimes follows sexual abuse. In one training for Spanish-speaking foster parents that I conducted, an experienced Latina foster mother said proudly that she had caught one of the girls in her home masturbating and told her that if she ever caught her doing that again she'd throw her out on the street. This woman cared deeply about the many foster children she had received in her home over the years, but had never learned a compassionate alternative to the punishing responses to sexual behavior with which she had been raised. Clearly, her response would shame the children in her care, and rather than helping them to resolve their sexual issues would most likely drive the behaviors underground.

Many cultures share the mistaken view that boys who have been abused sexually by men will become homosexuals as adults (Fontes, 1995a). There is no indication that sexual abuse will influence a boy's later sexual orientation (Arey, 1995). It is important for professionals to address this concern directly with families. Fathers, in particular, may become anxious about their son's sexual orientation and masculinity. It can be helpful to explain to parents and children who are old enough that no one entirely understands the development of sexual orientation. Many boys respond to being touched sexually by having an erection or even an orgasm because that is how boys are physiologically constructed. This can be compared to people startling when they hear a loud noise. This natural response does not indicate how a boy will choose to behave sexually as an adult. Parents who are concerned because their sons did not resist sexual abuse, delayed their disclosure, or participated in multiple incidents must be helped to understand that many factors, including coercion, shame, and threats, can contribute to boys keeping the secret of the abuse. Boys who are abused at a young age by men may become aware of the stigma attached to their victimization as they reach puberty and may need a new round of counseling at this point.

In my area, a young Latino boy was hit over the head with a brick and then sodomized. He sustained some disfigurement and mild brain damage as a result. His parents consoled themselves by saying, "At least no one could think that he was asking for it, that he was a *maricón* [faggot]." I worked with a Puerto Rican family where the father and older brothers of a boy who had been abused sexually by a man teased him mercilessly as a *maricón* due to the abuse he had suffered. The teasing soon spread, through friends of the boy's brothers, to the entire school, creating a living hell for this young man. The family was not psychologically minded and apparently had little notion of the possible long-term impact of such teasing. Several sessions of family therapy with a psychoeducational component permitted all the family members to discuss their feelings about the abuse, and then learn how they could support the young victim. The boy was able to get a fresh start in a new school.

Boys who have been sexually abused appear to engage in more sexual behaviors, such as masturbating, sexual play, and sexual aggression with younger children, than boys who have not been sexually abused, particularly between the ages of 7 and 12 (Friedrich et al., 1992). It is crucial, therefore, that clinicians explicitly address sexual issues in their work with boys who have been abused (Friedrich, 1995). This may be a delicate matter for families from cultures that rarely address sexual issues directly. Families may be eager to terminate services and put this chapter behind them. I recommend a matter-of-fact psychoeducational approach to the topic.

In addition to fears around homosexuality, many families fear that boys will become sexual offenders as a result of being victimized. They may need to be reassured that *most* men who were abused sexually do *not* offend against others, and that quality intervention can assist a boy in his recovery. Many victims grow up to be helpers: police, social workers, etc.

In sum, families of girl and boy victims of sexual abuse need to be helped to picture an optimistic future for their children in which the sexual abuse eventually becomes a mere footnote to an otherwise normal and positive life.

## Revictimization

In some cultures, when a girl is known to have been sexually abused, she has lost the special protective aura of virginity and is considered to be "fair game" for other men to try to seduce or even assault. There seems to be a notion that once she has been violated, she cannot be violated again. A number of studies have found that girls and women who have been sexually abused once are at greater risk for repeated sexual victimization in their child and adult years. Russell (1986) suggests that knowledge of prior victimization may disinhibit some offenders' abusive tendencies toward these girls: "Some people apparently find the information that a child has participated in a taboo sexual relationship exciting and provocative, regardless of the involuntary nature of the child's victimization" (p. 171). Russell suggests that victims are also at greater risk for further victimization because the attitude of blaming the victim "can serve as an ideological disinhibitor: 'She must have been asking for it' can easily turn into 'she's asking for it now too'" (p. 171).

Along the same lines, one Puerto Rican woman I interviewed described confiding in her pastor that her uncle was touching her inappropriately, "so then he started grabbing me and rubbing up against me, too." Even in situations where an offender does not know that a girl has been sexually abused, he may be able to detect indications of her shame, her low self-esteem, and her unrequited need for approval and affection, and then use these to exploit her sexually.

Grauerholz (2000) describes a variety of reasons why girls and women may be more likely to suffer further experiences of sexual assault following sexual abuse in childhood. These include continued exposure to the factors that put her at risk initially, lessened ability to detect danger, and use of substances that inhibit her ability to avoid dangerous situations or to escape from them. I believe that professionals rarely focus sufficiently with children and families on the need to prevent future victimizations; attending to the initial incident often seems to be more urgent and compelling.

Pearce and Pezzot-Pearce (1997) describe in some detail ways to work with children and families to avert future victimization without resorting to stifling efforts at overprotection. Often immigrant parents will respond to sexual assault by keeping their daughters as virtual prisoners in their homes. "You come straight home from school and don't talk to anyone!" These well-intentioned efforts to protect can make the child feel like she is being punished for her victimization. These are well-meaning attempts by parents to compensate for the feeling that they failed to protect their child adequately. The parents may need some assistance in developing a plan that balances the need for safety with their child's legitimate need to lead as normal a life as possible.

## Layers of Shame

Numerous ethnic minority writers have described feelings of shame related to their skin color, hair texture, eye shape, or social status. Several of these are described in Chapter 2. My mother, for instance, was ashamed of her long nose and her accent, which branded her as being from a working-class, immigrant, Polish Jewish family at a time when Jews were seen as foreign and dirty. Plastic surgery and diction lessons enabled her to avoid bias on these counts. She also deliberately studied the dress and habits of the upper social classes, and shaped herself carefully (she even learned to play tennis) so she could fit in with the ruling class. Many immigrants and members of ethnic minority groups cannot cast off the outer signs of their class or ethnic identity so easily (for instance, if their skin is not white, or if they don't have the income to get braces and attend to skin problems). While group identifiers are a source of pride at some moments, they can be a source of shame at others. "Rejection of who we are is a pressure we feel in all encounters," writes a Pakistani psychotherapist about the experience of "immigrant women of color" in Canada (Javed, 1995, p. 18).

Members of ethnic minority groups typically feel empowered by their identities in some contexts, and delighted to be from cultures that are distinct from the mainstream. However, most members of ethnic minority groups have also experienced moments when they were shamed for not conforming to the dominant ideal. I remember when my first boyfriend touched my kinky hair and said, "I thought girls' hair was supposed to be long and silky." An African American student told me about the first racial incident that she could remember, when another kindergartener refused to hold her hand because it was brown. These instances get tucked away into a well of shame inside members of oppressed groups. Additional shaming experiences, like sexual abuse or encounters with biased professionals, can bring this shame to the surface.

Let us consider all the layers of shame that might be experienced by a low-income African American woman who was abused sexually. Let's call her Angela. She has experienced the shame of her body being used by another for his pleasure, without regard for her will. She has experienced the shame of keeping the secret from members of her family, making her feel like she doesn't "belong" in her family. She has experienced the shame of being devalued by some members of the dominant group because of her race. Internalized racism may have contributed to her feeling ashamed of her skin tone or her hair among other African Americans, if she is considered either "too White" or "too Black." In some contexts, she may feel ashamed of being a woman in a society that clearly values men more than women. If she is a lesbian, she is a member of another stigmatized group. If she grew up speaking African American Vernacular English and never mastered Standard English, she may feel the shame of not knowing how to speak the language of those who hold power. Seeking help for sexual abuse, or being forced to accept social services, is apt to induce shame for her as well: she may have been told that "only crazy people go to shrinks" and only "bad families" need social workers. If the professional is White or is a man, she may feel particularly degraded by making herself vulnerable in the professional encounter. We need to understand and work through many layers of shame before we can begin to expect Angela to reveal herself to us.

To counteract shame, we must welcome all facets of Angela's self into our work together. By our attitude, we tell her that she is beautiful, she is intelligent, she is whole, and she will recover. We communicate our belief in her power. We interact with her so as to counteract her shame, and in no way contribute to it.

In a piece on a young Korean American, Kaya, who was drugged and sexually assaulted by her boss, Chan (1999) describes how Kaya felt that she had not only "lost face" through the assault, but how the recounting of the incident in therapy added another layer of shame. Chan writes that even as the young woman came to realize that she was not responsible for the assault, she still was unable to tell anyone in her family about the incident because that would have caused her—and the parents who had failed to protect her—to lose face. While acknowledging the concept of shame in Korean culture and its importance to the client, Chan reports encouraging her to "try on" the perspective of a victim from the dominant U.S. culture, to experiment with seeing herself as a wronged victim, and to consider—as an American woman might—seeking legal or professional support to charge her assailant with a crime (p. 82). Chan writes that she did not expect Kaya necessarily to engage in any of these activities, but that simply considering them might offer her some measure of relief from shame.

## COUNTERACTING SHAME

How can professionals help counteract the shame induced by child sexual abuse? It is important to remember that the shame has two components: the feeling of lack of *self*-worth and the feeling of lack of *social* worth. Separate steps may be required to counteract each of these two aspects of shame. Here are some brief tips, in addition to those included earlier in this chapter. These ideas are meant to be suggestive, rather than exhaustive, and their appropriateness with a given family or individual needs to be assessed carefully.

### Ideas for Working with Children

• Many children benefit from psychotherapy or psychoeducational groups with other children their age to reduce their sense of shame and isolation and to help them learn coping strategies.
• The special issue of the journal *Child Maltreatment* (Kolko & Feiring, 2002) that focuses on children's attributions about abuse is chock-full of suggestions for reducing shame for child victims of sexual abuse. In that issue Celano, Hazzard, Campbell, and Lang (2002) describe dozens of techniques using art, music, role playing, and talk therapy for changing the attributions in children of all ages. For instance, a child can create a "responsibility ruler" to measure out the relative responsibility of different people for his or her abuse.
• With children, family intervention is key. Children will decide what the abuse means to them based in large part on how the adults and other

children in their families respond. While this is true for all children, this may be especially true for children from immigrant families. Often immigrant families spend more time together than families from the dominant culture, and immigrant children may rely more on their families and less on their peers or other adults for social cues. Therefore, continual work with families of child sexual abuse victims will largely shape the child's long-term outcome.

## Ideas for Working with Adult Survivors

• Allow the client to tell her story again and again, if she wishes, and respond with acceptance and reassurance. Make clear that you are not shocked or repulsed by her story or by her.

• Allow the client to choose *not* to tell his story until he is ready, if he chooses to wait, indicating that you are ready to hear it when he is ready to tell it. Especially for clients from cultures that do not customarily rely on cathartic accounts of difficult events, the victim may not need to retell the story of the abuse to recover from it.

• Allow the client alternate means of telling her story if she does not want to express it to you verbally. For instance, some people would rather start by writing it down, or saying it aloud to themselves when alone, or saying it in their native language, even if they know the professional does not understand.

• Help the client obtain psychoeducational materials about sexual abuse. Useful resources include *Beginning to Heal* (Bass & Davis, 2003) and *Outgrowing the Pain* (Gil, 1988), both of which are also available in Spanish.

• Help the client imagine what he or she would like others to say or what should have been said when the abuse happened.

• Along with the client, design and implement a shame-releasing ritual that fits in with the client's culture. For instance, for a Jewish woman this might be a *mikvah*, a ritual bath, in which—in the presence of other women who care about her—she ritually washes off the influence of the abuse and is declared clean again. With Native American clients, rituals that "bring an individual back to harmony or balance with self, family, environment, and society" (DeBruyn, Chino, Serna, & Fullerton-Gleason, 2001, p. 96) may be helpful. These may include sweat lodges, healing circles, or chantways. Religious clients might welcome a ritual involving prayer. The timing of these rituals is important: they should not be implemented before the client is ready. A ritual implemented too early could contribute to premature closure, and might actually make a client feel ashamed of "not being over it already."

• Many clients find it helpful to move into an advocacy position in relation to others who have been affected by similar issues by writing an article or editorial on sexual abuse for a local newspaper, or by volunteering in a shelter for battered women, at a food pantry, or on a women's crisis hotline, for instance.
• Many clients find it helpful to participate in therapy groups. These groups can be specific for members of a particular ethnic or age group, or open to all adult victims.

## CONCLUDING THOUGHTS

Clearly, this chapter has not exhausted all there is to say about working with members of culturally diverse groups on issues of child sexual abuse. More information related to this topic is contained in each of the other chapters of this book, and much valuable work is listed in the References in the back. I hope that by contributing to the understanding of cultural aspects of shame in child sexual abuse, I have helped readers see ways to assist the diverse people affected by this problem.

### QUESTIONS TO THINK ABOUT AND DISCUSS

1. What are three ways cultural issues affect a victim's experience of child sexual abuse?

2. What would you say to parents who are concerned about the future of their 10-year-old daughter who has been raped? How would this vary according to the family's cultural group? (You may discuss members of one particular cultural group, if you wish.)

3. What would you say to parents who are concerned about the future of a 13-year-old boy who had been molested over a 1-year period by a male neighbor? How would this vary according to the family's cultural group?

4. Why is shame an important concept when considering child sexual abuse for members of minority cultural groups?

5. Discuss some ways that your own views of sexuality impact your handling (or future handling) of situations involving the sexual abuse of children.

# CHAPTER SEVEN

# Working with Interpreters in Child Maltreatment

> amid the noise of traffic and English, it was a silent world.
> —ALVAREZ (2004, p. 7)

This chapter discusses ways to maximize understanding and minimize hassles when working with foreign language interpreters in professional encounters related to child abuse and neglect. This information is designed for interpreters, for people who work in agencies that use interpreters, and for everyone who works with people with limited English proficiency. I use the term "interpreter" for those who convey the spoken word and the term "translator" for those who convey the written word, as is common practice in the field. I regret that this chapter does not discuss interpreting for people who are deaf; while many of the issues are similar, there are also significant differences that fall beyond the scope of this chapter.

Interpreters make it possible to listen to children and families who otherwise would be voiceless in the child welfare and criminal justice systems. High-quality interpretation allows us to obtain information to protect children and win convictions in court. High-quality interpretation allows us to gain families' confidence, reduce their isolation, understand their worldview, and provide them with services. Poor-quality interpretation leads to frustration for all involved, and can leave children even more vulnerable than before intervention.

Interpreters may be needed at many stages during a child abuse investigation and intervention. They are useful when child protective services interviews a child or family about the suspicion of child maltreatment;

when a more thorough and formal investigation is conducted through a children's advocacy center, medical office, or police department, with the goal of establishing a court case; when custody decisions are being investigated by the courts, child protective services, psychotherapists, or attorneys; and when children or families are receiving psychotherapeutic and other longer term services.

In children's advocacy center interviews where a one-way mirror is available, the interpreter can either sit behind the mirror and interpret for the team as an interview is conducted in the child's native language, or can sit in the interview room and interpret for an interviewer and child who do not speak the same language. Sometimes one interpreter will be needed in the room and another behind the mirror.

As far as I know, there is no research on the role of interpreters in child maltreatment investigations and interventions. We do not know how often interpreters are used, who is doing the interpreting, or anything about what really happens during these conversations. Often these conversations occur between people who are serving as an arm of governmental authority and control, such as law enforcement, child protective services, or the courts, and people who are economically and politically marginalized. We do not know if interpreters challenge the professionals, act as advocates or ambassadors for clients, or reinforce professionals' institutional authority. Davidson (2000) concluded in his research on interpreting in medical interviews that interpreters *cannot* be "neutral machines of semantic conversion" (p. 379), but rather are active participants in the process. Davidson quotes the head of interpreting services at a major hospital as saying, "Interpreters are the most powerful people in a medical conversation" (p. 379).

In his recorded interviews, Davidson found that interpreters edited and deleted sections of conversation, directed conversations, defined the problem at hand, made their own determinations about what was important and not important to mention, failed to communicate some portions of both physicians' and patients' conversation, shaped messages (rather than just conveying them), served as co-interviewers, and generally supported the professionals' goals (such as keeping interviews short) when they might be in conflict with the patients' interests (such as giving a full recounting of their symptoms and concerns). Perhaps most disturbingly, Davidson found that in most cases the interpreters "were neither trained extensively nor supported institutionally, and they performed their work in an ad-hoc vacuum of accountability" (p. 386) in regard to the quality of their interpretations. Regrettably, my experience indicates that most interpreters in child maltreatment work in similar, if not worse, conditions.

Given the remarkable lack of research on the role of interpreters and the process of interpreting in child maltreatment conversations, this chapter is based on research in related areas, conversations with interpreters and with those who train interpreters, conversations with child maltreatment professionals who have worked with interpreters, viewing of interpreted forensic interviews, and my own experiences in the field.

## WHEN TO USE AN INTERPRETER

People with limited English proficiency need to be informed about their right to utilize an interpreter. They need to be told that they may request an interpreter at any point in the provision of services, even if they initially decline one. Some clients will refuse an interpreter's services out of pride or out of a fear that they will not be taken seriously if they do not speak in English. Often, people who "get by" in English in most situations will be putting themselves at a great disadvantage if they do not avail themselves of an interpreter in child abuse interviews and interventions, where even the slightest misunderstanding could have life-changing repercussions (see Chapter 2).

Often professionals will assume clients do not need an interpreter because they seem able to express themselves well enough in English. However, as the conversations proceed and become more precise and emotionally laden, and as the clients become tired and possibly stressed, their English often deteriorates. It is one thing to be able to make small talk or to buy groceries in a second language (in this case, English). It is quite another thing to give and receive complex information with tremendous consequences in that second language.

## FINDING AN INTERPRETER

When an interpreter is needed, agencies should try to obtain the services of a professionally trained interpreter. Some states have court certification, medical certification, or other types of official certifications for interpreters, while others do not. In most situations that do not take place in court, a court-certified interpreter, who may be prohibitively expensive, is not necessary. However, if the material is going to be used in court, professionals should check with their local district attorney to determine the requirements in their jurisdiction (see Hardy, 1998, for an excellent series of tips on court interpreters in child witness cases). Even if a court-certified interpreter is not necessary, interpreters used for situations as important as child maltreatment interviews and other encounters should be professionally trained. Agencies need to maintain an extensive list of professionally trained interpreters to achieve coverage in a variety of languages; they should not wait until they are in the middle of a crisis before they seek an interpreter in a language that might be less common in their area.

The federal order on serving people with limited English proficiency allows for agencies to rely on qualified voluntary community interpreters who are bound by confidentiality agreements.[1] Several women's crisis centers in my area have banded together to establish an intensive training program for bilingual volunteers, in which they are taught to serve as interpreters. Many of these bilingual volunteers end up taking further training to learn to work on the hotline and attend to crises. Volunteers from dozens of languages have been trained and are available within 24 hours. Not only does this increase the women's centers' ability to serve immigrant communities, it also increases knowledge of the centers' services within those communities. The bilingual volunteer training program serves as a form of outreach.

Baker (1981) urges agencies to be especially cautious when employing interviewers who claim fluency in a variety of languages and who may exaggerate their fluency in their eagerness to obtain work. For instance, a Polish immigrant may claim to be able to interpret in Polish *and* Russian, although he possesses only rudimentary abilities in Russian. An interpreter should be able to demonstrate certification in the specific language in which he or she is going to interpret. When a certified interpreter cannot be found, Baker recommends that another interpreter or a bilingual professional interview the would-be interpreter in each of the languages required, to save later embarrassment and difficulties. This interview should not focus simply on language competency; it should also assess for the interpreter's knowledge of the cultural issues of the target population and some of the difficulties that might emerge in the interpreted conversation.

Some agencies rely on companies that provide telephone interpreting services. These services can either be contracted on a monthly basis or used spontaneously and paid for by the minute. Typically, the professional calls the service and asks for an interpreter who closely matches the client's needs (e.g., an interpreter who speaks Egyptian Arabic). The telephone interpreters can be patched in to interpret phone calls or can be used for in-person interviews and sessions. When using the phone service for in-person contacts, the professional and the client speak into a telephone and then the interpreter renders the speech into the other language through the phone. While this arrangement is far better than *no* interpreting, it can be confusing and alienating (particularly for children) and should be used only as a last resort. It can be hard for people to trust the confidentiality of

---

[1]See the U.S. Department of Health and Human Services, Office of Civil Rights (1998), *Guidance Memorandum on Prohibition against National Origin Discrimination: Persons with Limited English Proficiency.*

interpreters whom they cannot even see, and the conversation becomes highly unnatural.

Agencies need to think carefully before asking their multilingual professional staff to take on interpreting duties without additional training or compensation. For instance, in some police and social work departments, multilingual professionals are asked to interpret for their colleagues in addition to carrying their own full caseloads. This is an unfair burden that may hinder the quality of their work. First, while these professionals are apt to be qualified in their own areas, they have not necessarily been trained in interpreting—which is its own professional field. Second, their language skills may not be strong enough for them to serve as interpreters. (I know a Latino police officer whose Spanish is mediocre at best. He is frequently asked to interpret for his colleagues and is reluctant to tell his sergeant that he is unqualified to interpret or that he needs to take a Spanish class—he believes it would make him lose value in the department.) Third, unless they are being hired to interpret and are receiving a reduced caseload to compensate for the time they spend interpreting, professionals who are asked to interpret in addition to fulfilling their regular responsibilities are being forced to perform two jobs. This is a recipe for burnout and a poor outcome.

## INFORMAL INTERPRETERS

Agencies must avoid informal ad hoc interpreters—for example, people from the child's family, family friends, and others. As agencies scramble at the last minute to meet the needs of the diverse families in their areas, sometimes they rely on secretaries, janitors, siblings, and others to interpret for child abuse interviews. Battering men have being asked to interpret for their wives and children—even though this is an obvious conflict of interest. I have heard of the local Spanish teacher—known to virtually everyone in the school system—being asked routinely to interpret child abuse interviews in Spanish. When an interpreter is used, children and families have the sense that the ears that are *really* hearing them are those of the interpreter. Clients may not speak openly when a local teacher or other well-known community member is interpreting out of concern that everyone in the school or community will end up knowing their business.

It is problematic to use untrained interpreters because:

• An untrained interpreter might be too embarrassed or disturbed by the material to interpret accurately. (Recently, when a child began revealing the sexual part of an assault, the Portuguese interpreter in my area blushed, shook his head, and said he could not repeat what the child had said.)

• An untrained interpreter may want to help the child or the child's family to save face, thereby failing to interpret some of the more embarrassing or incriminating information. This may be just the information that we need most. For instance, a young Puerto Rican girl disclosed that the uncle with whom she was living had sexually molested her. In the interview with the detective, the informal interpreter said to the girl in Spanish, "Why don't you say it was just physical abuse and not sexual abuse? You can get out of his home that way, and he won't get into so much trouble."

• An untrained interpreter is more likely to embellish or delete information. This could be particularly problematic in a legal setting, where inconsistencies in testimony (that are actually a result of faulty interpretation) might jeopardize a case.

• Untrained, informal interpreters are likely to be familiar only with their own dialect of the language. A trained interpreter should be familiar with the way their language is spoken in a variety of countries. (For example, *coger* is a common word in Spanish but it means different things throughout the world. In some countries it is an everyday word meaning "to get," and in others it is a particularly crude word for sexual intercourse. A trained interpreter should not stumble over a word like this and should know about its dual meanings.)

• An untrained interpreter might unknowingly use regionally specific words or English words that would not be understandable to the client. For example, I witnessed a child abuse interview that was interpreted by a Puerto Rican social worker who had no training in interpreting and used "Spanglish" throughout the interview. Spanglish is a form of Spanish used by many Latinos in English-speaking countries. It uses a large number of words that have been "borrowed" from English and sometimes transformed into Spanish by adding on Spanish endings or pronunciation. This interpreter asked the child what she did for *el Easter* and instructed her to *eskipear* (skip) an item on a checklist. The child—who had recently immigrated from Central America—did not understand these words, which were actually adaptations of English. This same social worker interpreted the interviewer's question "Can you tell me the difference between the truth and a lie" by using the Puerto Rican word for fib, *un embuste*. When the girl looked back blankly, the interpreter said she did *not* know the difference, which was not the case at all. Rather, the girl did not recognize the Puerto Rican word.

• In a forensic interview, a client might make a statement that is disjointed, inaccurate, or doesn't make sense. An untrained interpreter may try to read the client's mind and piece together such incoherent statements into a coherent whole. A trained interpreter would be able to convey the competency and form of the client's statement—not just the content.

• An untrained interpreter may not know or follow the rules of keeping confidential what happens in child abuse interventions. Nothing will make a client clam up quicker than the perception that word is going to get around. A Chinese language interpreter in a hospital near me used to betray confidences in this way, saying to a patient in the emergency room, for instance, "You should stop by to see Wang on the third floor; he's in for a bad liver." The hospital could not understand why the Chinese patients would not talk freely until a Chinese-speaking nurse sat in on a conversation and they found out that the interpreter could not be trusted.

• There can also be problems of *perceived* confidentiality and multiple relationships. Even if the person interpreting does not actually betray confidences, the child or parent will worry about this possibility. Everyone knows one another in some small ethnic communities. Trained interpreters will be able to explain their role and the concept of confidentiality, and then briefly explain their professional commitment to confidentiality.

• An untrained interpreter who knows the family or who is a member of the family's place of worship or community might want to control what the victim says or might report it back to others. One would hope that a trained interpreter would be professional enough to understand and respect the ethical mandates of accuracy and confidentiality. After all, his or her livelihood depends on it.

Children should never be asked to interpret for other children or for adults in child maltreatment interviews. This demand would put inappropriate pressure on a child, who would then feel responsible for the outcome of the interview, and might—indeed—be blamed by the family if the outcome was not to their liking. In addition, the child might not have adequate vocabulary or understanding to convey sexual detail or complex legal or medical information.

## PREPARING INTERPRETERS

Ideally, interpreters used in child maltreatment interviews and interventions are professionally trained, certified, and familiar with child maltreatment issues. In practice today this is often not the case, as agencies scramble to get conversations interpreted using whatever resources they have on hand. This section describes some of the orientation that nonprofessional interpreters may need before working on issues of child maltreatment. Much of this advice would be unnecessary and might actually be insulting to a professional interpreter. Readers need to use their judgment with each interpreter to see how much advice and guidance is necessary.

The children's advocacy center Corner House, in Minneapolis, provides required training for all interpreters who will be used in child abuse interviews. While this is certainly ideal, until your agency establishes such a program you may at least want to have a checklist you can review with interpreters before using their services, to make sure you have discussed all relevant information. The information that should be covered in such a preparatory discussion is outlined below.

The interviewer should meet the interpreter before the child or family walks in, and ask if he or she has any questions. The interpreter's name, qualifications, and contact information should be recorded. The interpreter needs to be reminded that confidentiality is of the utmost importance, and should be asked to read carefully and sign a pledge of confidentiality in which he or she promises not to speak about the interview or reveal the identity of the child or the family. The interpreter should be asked to discuss questions about confidentiality with the interviewer before the interview begins. Where relevant, the interpreter should be informed that there is some possibility that he or she will be asked to testify in court.

The interpreter should be asked to inform the interviewer immediately if he or she discovers that he or she knows the child's family or the child, so the interviewer can decide how to proceed. (In some cases, even where the interpreter has a prior contact with the family, an explanation of the interpreter's role and pledge of confidentiality will be sufficient to allay concerns and the session can proceed. In other situations, another interpreter may need to be called in.) If the child or family has had previous social contact with the interpreter, they may be evasive or overly polite and deny problems, difficult feelings, or sensitive issues.

We should tell interpreters about the nature of the interview or intervention we are undertaking, and help them understand that the interpreting needs to be done with more precision than in most other situations. For instance, interpreting for a standard medical exam might not require the same attention to careful phrasing because concerns about leading the interviewee would not have the same importance. Inform the interpreter that interviewers have to be careful about how they phrase questions and so they may sometimes ask questions in a way that seems funny, awkward, or indirect. It's important to instruct the interpreter not to rephrase any questions, but still to speak in a way that will be comprehensible to the client.

Baker (1981), in describing a court hearing, cautions against interpretation that overemphasizes exactness over understanding:

> The judge asked the [unaccompanied refugee minor] youths through an interpreter if they "agreed to being placed under the custody and guardianship of the agency and to follow the reasonable directions thereof." It was later discovered that the interpreter's close translation of this question had led the youths to believe they had been placed into slavery. (p. 392)

In other words, interpreters should stick closely to the language used, and at the same time ensure that the *meaning* of the statements is conveyed.

The interpreter should be asked to assure completeness in their work by not leaving out details that may at first seem unimportant. The interpreter should also be informed that if the client answers in partial sentences, in a confusing way, or in baby talk, these answers should be communicated in the manner in which they were stated, and not changed, clarified, or improved. The interpreter should not guess what the client meant but rather should repeat in English precisely what the client said. The interviewer needs to be told if the client's speech is confusing in some way. A trained interpreter will ask for a moment to give an "aside" during an interview, to inform the interviewer of some irregularity in the client's speech that otherwise may not be clear. For example, if the client has a notable stutter; exhibits articulation difficulties due to overmedication or another problem; appears to be in an altered state; or has other peculiarities that may be lost in the interpretation, the interpreter should convey this information to the interviewer since it might affect both the quality of the interpretation and the line of questioning (Ilia Cornier, private communication, March 21, 2004).

Interpreters should be informed that sometimes during interviews children will reveal that nothing harmful has happened, and conversely that sometimes clients talk about acts that are painful to hear about and repeat. They may talk about getting hurt in ways that are hard for the interpreter to imagine or believe, and that might make the interpreter feel sad or angry. The interpreter should be instructed to stay as neutral as possible and to avoid showing through manner or facial expressions that he or she may be upset, angry, or disgusted, or that he or she may disbelieve the client.

The interpreter should also be informed that the interviewer or the client (even a child) may use words that the interpreter is uncomfortable saying—slang words or sexual words, for instance. The interpreter should be asked to stick closely to the words that are used and try to put aside feelings of embarrassment. The interpreter should be instructed to try to use the same kind of words the interviewer and the client use. That is, if the client says the word "dick" in his or her first language, the interpreter should not substitute the more formal word "penis" but should try to use a similar kind of slang term.

## CULTURAL ASIDES AND OTHER REASONS
## TO PAUSE AN INTERVIEW

The interpreter serves as a kind of cultural bridge from the interviewer to the client and back. For instance, a Puerto Rican client may say something about his *padrino*. Rather than simply translating this term as "godfather" and moving on, the interpreter may want to briefly inform the interviewer that typically the role of godfather is an important one in Puerto Rican families.

In the course of an interview or other intervention, the professional may ask questions that could be offensive. Most professionals appreciate it when an interpreter informs them if this is a problem in a cultural aside. For instance, in trying to learn about a Japanese family, an interviewer might ask a parent questions about abuse in his or her own childhood. It might be helpful for the interpreter to tell the interviewer that the parent is not likely to answer this question truthfully before a relationship and context have been established, rather than allowing the interviewer to proceed with what will be considered offensive questioning. This added cultural information is far preferable to what often occurs: the interpreter fails to ask the potentially offensive questions and then fails to inform the interviewer of this omission.

The interpreter should be instructed to stop the interviewer if he or she needs to ask a question or to clarify a concept. If there is a concept that cannot be translated easily into English or into the other language, the interpreter should inform the interviewer. Similarly, if the interpreter does not understand a word because it is in a different dialect or for some other reason, the interviewer should be informed. This can be tricky because interpreters often need to give their best guess as to the meaning of a word as used by a particular client in a particular context. (For instance, in recounting sexual abuse in Spanish a client who uses the word *leche*, which literally means "milk," is apt to mean "ejaculate" or "cum" rather than the dairy product.) However, even when using his or her best professional judgment, the interpreter can still make mistakes. If the client uses a word which is unfamiliar to the interpreter (e.g., a special word for a body part), the interpreter can give the word in its original form to the interviewer and explain that he or she is not sure of its meaning. Then the interviewer can ask the child for clarification (e.g., perhaps by using an anatomical diagram), as would be done in an interview conducted in English.

Also, if the interpreter believes there is something wrong with the quality of the interpretation—and that this is such a big problem that the interview will not be accurate—the interviewer should be informed right away. For instance, sometimes Portuguese speakers are asked to interpret for interviews with Cape Verdeans (or French speakers with Haitians, or Spanish speakers with indigenous people of the Americas who do not speak Spanish). When he or she gets to the interview, the interpreter may discover that the client only speaks a little Portuguese, but mostly speaks Creole. Cape Verdean Creole contains some Portuguese words, but not enough to render an entire interview.

Sometimes a client is not verbal in any language because of a hearing, speech, or cognitive impairment. This may not become apparent until the client is approached in his or her first language. If the interviewer needs to establish an urgent safety plan for that day, then a less-than-ideally interpreted interview may be adequate for that day, while a better one is scheduled for a later date. However, if the interview is a formal forensic interview necessary to gather complete information for court, then a less-than-ideal interpretation should be rejected and the interview delayed until an interpreter who is better suited to the circumstances can be found.

## THE INTERPRETER'S ROLE

Some interpreters hope to establish an intimate and supportive relationship with a child or family, and to serve almost as a cultural broker or mediator. It is common in a court setting for interpreters to meet briefly with clients before the session begins to say, essentially:

> "I am so-and-so. I will be interpreting for you today in court. Anything you say to me I will be repeating in English to the person who is questioning you. If you try to ask me something directly, I will repeat it to the person who is interviewing you. Please do not think I am being unfriendly if I do not respond to you directly. My job here is just to help you understand everything that is being said to you, and help the person who is speaking to you understand everything you say. I am also going to ask that only one person speak at a time, so I can make sure I can hear each person clearly. I have promised confidentiality. That means that I will not repeat what you tell me to people who are not involved in your case. If we see each other in another situation sometime, you don't have to worry. I am a professional interpreter and will keep secret what you say. Do you have any questions?"

Professional interpreters find that this kind of brief introduction helps the client understand the interpreting process. Forensic interviewers sometimes prefer to have this introduction take place on camera or in the official interview room so that it becomes part of the official record.

Other than this brief introduction, the interpreter should not say anything to the client that the interviewer has not said. The interpreter should not reassure the client, ask the client if he or she is telling the truth, or give an opinion about what may have happened. The interpreter should not influence the client by suggesting an action to take or what to say. If the client asks the interpreter a question, the interpreter should convey that question to the interviewer so he or she can reply.

An interpreter should be as unobtrusive as possible. While the interpreter can be friendly, the interpreter should not try to make a connection with the client—that is the interviewer's job. In general, during an interview the interpreter *should not* seek out eye contact with the client. The interpreter's job is just to let the client and the interviewer communicate.

Interpreters should maintain a professional demeanor at all times. They should not give out their phone numbers to clients, establish a relationship with a client outside the professional situation, provide transportation to a client in their own cars, or accept gifts from clients. Any of these actions could compromise their neutrality and—by implication—hinder the success of a court case. These informal contacts could also make the interpreter aware of personal information relevant to a client's case, information that had not been revealed in the professional setting. For instance, Baker (1981) describes an interview in which a Vietnamese youth swore an interpreter to secrecy before revealing that he was planning to run away from his guardian. This was, of course, extremely awkward.

## THE INTERPRETED CONVERSATION

Interpreting between languages is more difficult when the languages and cultures are especially far apart in their concepts, structure, and origin. For example, Chinese and English share fewer concepts than German and English. But even in languages that share similar origins, misunderstandings frequently occur. Sometimes bilingual speakers "code switch" or use words and concepts from one language in another. This can make interpreting extremely difficult. For instance, when asked what happened next, a young Puerto Rican girl might respond, "*Me molestó.*" In Spanish, this means "*X* bothered me," without being clear who did the bothering (no pronoun was used). However, if the girl speaks some English, she might be using the word *molestar* in the English, sense, meaning "to molest." (In this case *molestar/molest* is a false cognate, a word that *sounds like* a word in the other language, but has a different meaning.) The problem of the missing pronoun remains—the girl could be referring to any person, man, woman, or child—

as having bothered or molested her. An interpreter must make a multitude of fast-paced decisions to render accurately this seemingly simple sentence of just two words.

We should avoid using technical or legal jargon, such as "lascivious intent," or abbreviations, such as "perp," or "CPS," in conversations that are being interpreted unless there is some particular reason why the technical term is required (e.g., if someone is being charged, they should know the particular charge and be given an explanation of that charge). Additionally, we need to be aware that careful interpretation may require using long explanatory phrases to convey something that is a simple concept in English. Conducting an interview through an interpreter will take longer than conducting an interview in one language only. We should schedule longer blocks of time (if the client can tolerate it) for those sessions that are interpreted. Nevertheless, if the interviewer and the interpreter work well together, they can establish a good rhythm.

Interviewers should do their best to assure that acoustics in the interview room are conducive to interpreting. Hearing well is key to being able to interpret. Professionals should do their best to eliminate extraneous noises such as loud fans or background music.

In adversarial situations, such as when an accusation is made against an alleged perpetrator of violence, different people should interpret for the victim and the accused to keep each testimony as "pure" as possible. A child, in particular, who sees a person interpreting for the accused, and thereby speaking "in the voice" of the accused, may be inhibited about speaking freely with that interpreter present.

The interviewer should speak as if he or she is talking directly to the client. For example, he or she should say, "What did you have for breakfast this morning?," addressing the client, rather than saying to the interpreter, "Ask her what she had for breakfast this morning." And when the client speaks, the interpreter should speak in the client's voice, also using the first person, as in "I ate bread," rather than "She says she ate bread." This preserves the immediacy of the relationship and avoids confusion (Bradford & Muñoz, 1993).

Languages are filled with metaphoric speech that can sometimes lead to cross-cultural misinterpretation. In general, interpreters are trained to find an equivalent English-language expression for the expression in the original language. That is, if a client says, *"Me costó un ojo de la cara"* (literally, "It cost me an eye from my face"), that should be interpreted as "It cost me a mint." In practice, many metaphoric expressions do not have an exact equivalent in both languages. Moreover, even if they do, they are often hard to think of in the moment. Interpreters will typically say "She used a metaphoric expression meaning that it was very expensive" to interpret the above expression.

Rather than working as cotherapists or cointerviewers, the professional and the interpreter in child abuse situations try to work as one person, with the interpreter conveying the personal style and approach of the professional. According to Baker (1981), "A gentle statement must be translated gently, for example; a confrontation must be translated as such; and a supportive statement must reflect warmth in its content" (p. 393).

In an interview the participants should be positioned so that the interviewer can establish a connection with the client. The interpreter should probably sit to the side of and slightly behind the client. The interviewer should look at the client, not at the interpreter. Although it may seem funny at first, the interviewer should listen to the interpreter without looking at him or her. If the interviewer focuses on the client, smiles at the client, speaks to the client directly, and makes occasional eye contact with the client, it will be easier for the client to feel connected.

If an agency relies on the same interpreter regularly, this interpreter should have the opportunity to benefit from supervision about his or her interpreting. If the interview or intervention is recorded electronically, then another professional interpreter should be asked to review the quality of the recorded interpretation (respecting the confidentiality of the original intervention, of course). Or another interpreter could be asked to sit in on or observe the interpreting from time to time. This peer supervision is similar to that received by all professionals, and should be conducted in a spirit of cooperation and helpfulness. Formal or informal peer supervision of this kind helps interpreters keep their skills honed and their work fresh and interesting.

## Simultaneous versus Consecutive Interpreting

In simultaneous interpretation, the interpreter listens and speaks at virtually the same time rather than waiting for pauses to repeat what he or she remembers. Some writers suggest that simultaneous interpretation improves the accuracy, speed, and naturalness of interpretations (Bradford & Muñoz, 1993). However, simultaneous interpretations require that two people speak at the same time (e.g., the interpreter and the client). This produces a confusing record, and makes it virtually impossible for a stenographer to record the conversation or to produce a written transcript of a recorded conversation. In general, in question-and-answer situations where the conversation is either recorded or documented (as is usually the case in child abuse interviews and interventions), consecutive interpretation is preferred. In consecutive interpretation, the client and professional are asked to speak clearly in relatively short utterances, pausing between each utterance to allow the interpreter to render the speech into the other language. Only one person speaks at a time. While this is slower than simultaneous interpretation, it may be less confusing to all parties—since only one voice is heard at a time.

## Interpreting for Children and for People with a Low Level of Intelligence

An interpreter may need to adjust his or her practice when interpreting for a young child or a person with a low level of intelligence or certain kinds of mental illness. A 5-year-old, for instance, may be confused by an interpreter who has just introduced herself as "Ms. Jones, the interpreter," and then immediately interprets the interviewer's speech (in the first person), saying, "I'm Caroline Thomas, I'm a doctor, and I have a few questions for you today." When working with people who would be confused by this constant switching of person, interpreters may choose, instead, to say, "The doctor wants to know. . . . " In other words, the interpreter's goal is to convey conversation in the clearest way possible. Occasionally this demands straying from standard interpreting practice.

Additionally, when working with a young child, the interpreter will need to be a full human being. The child may feel like he or she is speaking to the interpreter—who may be more likely to be from the same ethnic group and is more likely to understand the cultural norms than the interviewer. When working with a young child, the interpreter will probably want to be warm and affectionate and inspire the child's trust, rather than coolly withholding warmth and eye contact. An experienced court interpreter, Ilia Cornier (personal communication, March 22, 2004) described to me interpreting for a child victim in a brutal rape case in superior court. When she met the child, she asked him where he wanted her to sit. The child requested that she sit with him in the witness box, and in the end crawled into her lap to give testimony.

## THE EMOTIONAL COST OF INTERPRETING IN CHILD ABUSE SITUATIONS

Interpreting well is hard work. The interpreter must be completely fluent in both languages and tuned in to differences in word usage. He or she must listen, speak, and translate all at once. Additionally, since emotional rapport and empathy is crucial, the interpreter tries to convey the same feelings and use the same intonation as the people being interpreted. This requires not just linguistic dexterity but emotional dexterity as well.

Interpreting in child abuse interviews and other encounters involving interpersonal violence can be especially grueling emotionally. A highly experienced court interpreter told me recently about how she was shaking after interpreting the victim impact statement of a sadistic rape. These cases are difficult for all of us to hear, but we must remember that the interpreter is using the word "I" and speaking in the first person throughout, as if he or she is the victim, or in some cases the defendant. The interpreter is expected to stay neutral, and therefore must constantly repress any sign of partiality to one side or the other. The interpreter may be aware that certain unstated bits of information would be helpful, and yet it is not his or her role to seek out or to convey this extra information. Typically, court interpreters do not have mental health training, do not belong to a supportive team with whom they can debrief, and may be expected to move directly from one tense and traumatic case to another without pause (Ilia Cornier, personal communication, February 2004).

Children's advocacy centers, child protective services agencies, and others who frequently rely on interpreters for help with difficult material may try to cultivate a group of interpreters with whom they work regularly, who are familiar with the system. It may be important to hold a brief debriefing (or postinterview review; see Freed, 1988) with the interpreter after a particularly difficult session. This will provide humane relief for the interpreter and make him or her less likely to discuss the case with friends or coworkers. The interpreter who feels valued and like part of a team effort will be more likely to return on future days to interpret other difficult interviews. This debriefing will also serve as a forum to check the accuracy of the interpretation. Although the interpreter may be eager to learn more about the process and what will happen next, it would be inappropriate for other professionals to discuss anything specific to the case beyond that which took place during the interpreted conversation.

This postinterview discussion can also afford an opportunity for the interpreter to convey information that may not have been conveyed during the interview regarding peculiarities of the client's accent, articulation, affect, or anything else that may be of interest.

## CONCLUDING THOUGHTS

We do not know how using an interpreter shapes the way we see the people with whom we are working, and how they see us. Davidson (2000) found that interpreters in medical interviews often thwarted rather than facilitated the parts of the conversation that were initiated by the patients. In particular, the interpreters failed to communicate the patients' questions. Sometimes the interpreters answered the patients' questions themselves, and sometimes the interpreters just ignored the questions. Davidson speculates that these failures increase the likelihood that the patients will be seen as "passive" by their service providers (p. 391). Clearly, also, the patients were not receiving the most informed answers to their questions. In addition, the physicians were not becoming aware of the patients' concerns. If the same sorts of failures occur in interpreted child maltreatment conversations, as I expect they do, this could be serious, indeed.

Child maltreatment professionals are entirely dependent on interpreters in situations where their services are used. If a conversation is interpreted inaccurately—either intentionally or unintentionally—the interviewer is unlikely to find out. It is crucial, therefore, that child maltreatment professionals find, train, and cultivate relationships with competent interpreters who understand and respect the boundaries of their role.

## QUESTIONS TO THINK ABOUT AND DISCUSS

1. Discuss ways the agencies in your area can go about improving their access to competent interpreters. Which immigrant communities are most in need of services?

2. Is your agency providing the same quality services to people who have limited English proficiency as they are to others? If not, what else should be done?

3. If you have worked with an interpreter in a child maltreatment situation, describe a time when it worked particularly well. What made it work well?

4. If you have worked with an interpreter in a child maltreatment situation, describe a time when it worked poorly. What was problematic about it?

5. What would it feel like to be 8 years old and be asked a lot of personal questions by an adult in a language you don't understand, and then hear the questions again in your own language? What might make this process easier?

# CHAPTER EIGHT

# Child Maltreatment Prevention and Parent Education

In this chapter I discuss ways to improve the ability of child maltreatment prevention programs and parent education to reach immigrant and ethnic minority families. Like most others who work in this field, I would like to see an end to the need for our services one day in the future. Clearly, while investigation, legal prosecution, and victim support are important, the ultimate goal is to prevent abuse from occurring. To be effective, the preventive efforts must fit the clients' cultures.

I served on the advisory committee of a research group that was investigating the effectiveness of a home visiting program to reduce child maltreatment among young first-time parents. Private agencies held local contracts to implement this statewide initiative. Each agency was charged with meeting the needs of the diverse ethnic communities in their areas. As a committee, we were puzzled by the difficulty several agencies were having in recruiting immigrant participants into the program—despite a high immigrant presence in their cities and towns. One day I happened to be listening to a Spanish-language radio station while driving through a heavily Latino city and heard a representative from a local agency make a recruitment plea for participants. She spoke in Spanish, in the most condescending terms, about how an agency worker would be willing to go into the home of a poor girl who happened to find herself pregnant and needed some help to make sure she wouldn't abuse her baby. She stated that some young parents actually kill their children because of incompetence!

Part of the answer to the recruitment difficulty immediately became evident: lack of cultural sensitivity. In this case, the agency was making an effort to do outreach to the Latino community, but its spokesperson on the radio seemed to be poorly trained and supervised. She was making an "appeal" for participants in the most unappealing way, and in a manner that would surely alienate the young Latina mothers she wanted to reach. As is often the case, if the bilingual worker's supervisors did not speak the second language, the worker had probably received inadequate or no supervision regarding her outreach in that language. Her appeal emphasized the mothers' potential deficits—not an approach likely to attract eager participants.

## CHILD MALTREATMENT PREVENTION

Prevention is the key to ending child maltreatment. Most child abuse professionals will now say with confidence, "Prevention works." Or, more accurately, "High-quality prevention programs work." The results of school-based sexual abuse prevention programs are promising (see Plummer, 2004), and both center-based and home-based abuse and neglect prevention programs have had a range of positive outcomes (Daro, 2003). No one program can reach all potential caretakers adequately. For this reason, prevention professionals recommend a variety of services in many formats to reach different audiences (Daro & Cohn Donnelly, 2002).

Despite their success, however, prevention programs are poorly funded and often among the first to be cut when budgets are tight. While the criminal justice system has a vested interest in apprehending criminal offenders, and government officials have a vested interest in funding caseworkers to avoid embarrassing headlines about dead or missing children in the child welfare system, no similar constituency exists to advocate for giving child abuse *prevention* a high priority. Child welfare agencies—typically severely underfunded—have trouble justifying taking dollars away from direct casework and applying them to prevention. Prevention remains a relatively impoverished area within the child abuse field, and it claims but a miniscule amount of public funding as compared to child abuse intervention, criminal prosecutions, and defense against other dangers.[1]

### The Case for Cultural Competency

This sad state of affairs seems even sadder when we consider the communities whose members/residents are most likely to get caught up in the child protection system: the poor, immigrants, and disproportionate numbers of African American and Native American families. Unfortunately, the advocacy groups for ethnic populations, such as La Raza or the National Asso-

---

[1]For an excellent general review of prevention programs, including a discussion of programs that work, see, U.S. Department of Health and Human Services, Administration for Children and Families (2003).

ciation for the Advancement of Colored People (NAACP), do not generally advocate for ethnic families impacted by child maltreatment because they tend to steer away from issues that carry any social stigma (such as child abuse and AIDS). So the result of not preventing child abuse is felt disproportionately in poor and ethnic minority communities, as more children are injured physically and emotionally, more families torn asunder, more children placed in foster care or juvenile detention, and more adults incarcerated for preventable acts.

A recent survey of the literature reveals a glaring lack of information about how to achieve cultural competency in child abuse prevention. Discussions of child abuse prevention typically call for an expansion of "culturally sensitive programs." Plummer (2004) reports that more sexual abuse prevention programs have "culture specific program components" today than 10 and 20 years ago. However, there is little available literature on what a "culturally sensitive program" or a "culture specific program" might look like. This chapter fills some of that gap.

To be most effective, prevention programs must target the specific needs of the populations they are meant to influence (Thomas, 1998). Research and public health initiatives aimed at curbing the spread of AIDS, for instance, include a myriad of programs targeting the specific circumstances of gay men (Rosser, Coleman, & Ohmans, 1993), Latino farm workers (Magana, 1991), high school students, drug users (Schilling et al., 1989), rural populations (Rounds, 1986), Asian and Pacific Islander communities (Yep, 1994), and so on. Similarly, programs aimed at reducing substance abuse target separately the specific needs of different age, gender, and cultural groups.

In contrast, most child abuse prevention programs remain remarkably "generic," meaning they are usually developed by and for members of the majority racial group (White) without regard for cultural differences. Although discussions of child maltreatment prevention frequently bemoan this lack of culture-specific programs and the lack of research on the success of prevention efforts according to ethnic culture, change in this area remains slow. Deborah Daro (2003), who has focused her distinguished career on child abuse prevention, reminds us that "prevention is often about building a relationship, not simply about delivering a product" (p. 4). These key relationships between caretakers and prevention professionals will form *only* when families are approached in ways that fit their culture and circumstances.

## Primary, Secondary, and Tertiary Prevention

Prevention programs may be grouped into primary, secondary, and tertiary prevention. *Primary prevention programs* are universal and directed at the general population. They attempt to stop maltreatment from occurring. Typically, they raise the awareness of the general public, service providers, and decision makers about child maltreatment. Primary prevention programs include "public service announcements that encourage positive parenting; parent education programs and support groups that focus on child development and age-appropriate expectations and the roles and responsibilities of parenting; family support and family strengthening programs that enhance the ability of families to access existing services and resources and support interactions among family members; and public awareness campaigns that provide information on how and where to report suspected child abuse and neglect" (U.S. Department of Health and Human Services, Administration for Children and Families, 2003).

Primary prevention programs are advantageous because they reach all parents, potential parents, and interested others, and because their very universality means there is no stigma attached to their use. In much of Europe, Australia, and New Zealand, for example, home health visitors routinely visit *all* new mothers shortly after the birth of their first child (Kamerman & Kahn, 1993). This may be seen as a primary prevention program, and has been found to reduce child maltreatment. General public education campaigns can achieve the primary prevention goal of preventing abuse by encouraging caretakers to care for children better, avoid abusive behaviors (such as shaking babies), and seek professional assistance. They have been found to reduce both corporal punishment and verbal aggression in disciplining children (Daro & Gelles, 1992). They also appear to make parents and other caretakers more open to other kinds of family interventions, such as home visiting (Daro & Cohn Donnelly, 2002). General public education campaigns can also achieve the secondary and tertiary prevention goals of making it easier for children and adults to recognize and seek help for child victimization (Daro, 1994).

The disadvantage of primary prevention is that by spreading resources widely and universally, reduced resources are available for the concentrated services required by at-risk populations. While it is true that a little can help a lot of people, it is also true that some people need more than a little help.

*Secondary prevention programs* target populations that are considered to have special risk factors associated with child maltreatment, such as young maternal age, poverty, parental substance abuse, or child disabilities. These programs may also be directed to neighborhoods that have high rates of risk factors or high rates of child maltreatment. Secondary prevention programs include support groups for stressed parents, parent education programs targeted to teen or substance-abusing parents, home visiting programs in poor neighborhoods with a high rate of child maltreatment, psychotherapy and respite care for parents of children with special needs, and family centers that provide information and referrals to families living in low-income neighborhoods (U.S. Department of Health and Human Services, Administration for Children and Families, 2003). As you can see, the same program (e.g., home visiting, parenting groups) can be considered either primary or secondary prevention, depending on whether it is universal or targeted.

*Tertiary prevention programs* are activities focused on reducing the negative consequences of maltreatment where it has already occurred and preventing its recurrence. Examples of tertiary prevention programs include family therapy or intensive casework focused on child maltreatment issues, psychotherapy groups for child victims or adult survivors of sexual abuse, intensive family intervention services or parent aides for families involved with child protective services, family violence response teams (Delson, Gaba, & Walker, 2003), and court-mandated anger management or parenting classes for physically abusive parents. Culturally competent and culturally specific tertiary prevention services such as psychotherapy are discussed elsewhere in this book, and parenting groups will be discussed at the end of this chapter.

## Targeting Prevention to Ethnic Communities: Challenges and Promises

Primary, secondary, and tertiary prevention programs can all be implemented in ways that are culturally competent. Often the first goal of prevention efforts is to inform people about child maltreatment and encourage them to acknowledge that child abuse occurs in their midst. This can be particularly difficult for members of stigmatized groups:

> Significant segments of the African American community have traditionally taken a twofold thematic variation of "see no evil, hear no evil." On one hand, sexually abusing children is something other ethnic groups do. On the other hand, if, in fact, African Americans do engage in incestuous acts or other sexually abusive behavior with children, it is not to be talked about because it is thought that acknowledging sexual child abuse will be used in some damnable way to further exclude African Americans from the American mainstream. (Abney & Priest, 1995, p. 11)

While this paragraph concerns African Americans and sexual abuse specifically, I have heard similar sentiments expressed by members of various other ethnic communities concerning all kinds of family violence. For this reason, an agency that wishes to target prevention efforts to members of a specific ethnic community may be received skeptically at best, as leaders and members of that community wonder, "Why are you targeting *us*?"

and "How is this going to be used against us?" Thus it would be important to convey repeatedly a message such as: "Our agency has discovered we have not been successful at reaching the Vietnamese families who live in this city with our child abuse prevention messages. We do *not* believe that child abuse is more common among Vietnamese families, but we do want to correct our failure to provide services to our Vietnamese neighbors." This kind of message conveys respect for the community and may help relieve some of its initial suspicion. (Other factors regarding the acceptance of services in ethnic communities are discussed below and in Chapters 1, 2, and 9.)

## Public Awareness Campaigns

Agencies that hope to work with members of ethnic minority communities will need to reach out into those communities in every possible way. Everywhere we see commercial advertisements, that's where our ads should also be. Agencies may have to seek corporate sponsors for those spaces. Via public service announcements in buses, subways, telephone booths, and highway billboards; through television commercials; on the Internet; on supermarket register tapes, in telephone books, and on milk cartons—we should be letting people know about child development, about norms for attentive, nonviolent child rearing, and about available community services. Our fliers should be handy in the bathrooms of religious institutions, school hallways, guidance counselors' offices, medical offices, and hospital waiting rooms. We should hang posters and place fliers about our services in ethnic supermarkets, nail salons, automotive repair shops, bars, and beauty parlors.

Some AIDS educators have successfully used beauticians, manicurists, bartenders, and taxi drivers as outreach workers on AIDS prevention. These professionals have gladly attended trainings so that they could learn more about halting the spread of AIDS. Child abuse professionals could use the same approach. We should set up child abuse awareness weeks, or healthy children months, with the specific aim of reaching communities that we don't serve well enough now. We need to ask the spiritual leaders in ethnic communities—priests, ministers, rabbis, imams, and other clergy—to discuss various kinds of child abuse and to distribute information about available services. We need to get local radio and TV newscasters to run stories about our activities and successes. Only through these efforts will underserved populations come to know about and trust people who work in child welfare. We should facilitate focus groups in these ethnic communities to figure out the needs of the specific communities and the sources of information they are most likely to trust (Fontes, 1997).

I helped STOP IT NOW!, a child sexual abuse prevention organization, design focus groups to be conducted in Philadelphia to determine the sexual abuse prevention needs in African American and Latino communities (Fontes et al., 2001). When asked about disseminating messages to their community, participants from both groups recommended getting information out to the public through announcements and information on the radio and in community newspapers; educational materials and sessions in schools, stores, childcare centers, 12-step meetings, block parties, health fairs, and recreation centers; working with visible and trusted community organizations; and posting flyers in public places such as bus stops and bus stations.

Latino participants also talked about the importance of the personal connection. They encouraged one-on-one education, including home visits. They pointed out that many city blocks have block representatives as part of citizens' patrol groups, and noted that these neighborhood leaders would be good people to target to teach and then disseminate information about child abuse. Some Latino participants indicated they would be comfortable conducting door-to-door education campaigns. Perhaps this possibility is uniquely suited to some Latino communities where there is a tradition of in-person contact and door-to-door evangelizing and sales. In these focus groups, Latinos and African Americans suggested setting up circles of chairs in parks and other places where people congregate during the summer, serving lemonade, and providing information on child abuse prevention.

## Sexual Abuse Prevention

Preventing sexual abuse is somewhat different from preventing other kinds of child maltreatment. Sexual abuse differs from other forms of child abuse in many ways, including the fact that approximately 50% of the offenders are persons other than the victim's parents, compared to 10% for physical abuse and 8% for neglect (Jones, Finkelhor, & Kopiec, 2001). Sexual abuse seems more criminal and highly stigmatized, whereas other forms of child maltreatment sometimes seem like "accidents" or unfortunate consequences of generally accepted actions (e.g., spanking a child too hard). Plummer (2004) describes sexual abuse prevention as more ideologically charged than other forms of child maltreatment prevention:

> Preventing [sexual] abuse necessitates changing attitudes in a society where often children are seen as property, women as sex objects, pornography as harmless, sexual crimes as uncontrollable, the effects of abuse as negligible,

the extent of abuse as insignificant, and unwanted touch as a normal part of life. Preventing sexual abuse calls into question many of our unexamined values. (p. 290)

Prevention efforts against physical abuse and neglect usually focus on altering problematic parenting practices. They have traditionally targeted caretakers. On the other hand, prevention efforts against sexual abuse have traditionally aimed at increasing children's ability to detect suspicious behavior, to resist attempted assaults, and to tell about them (Daro & Cohn Donnelly, 2002). Recently, public awareness campaigns about sexual abuse have also targeted the general public concerning ways to protect children, detect risk, and report suspicions (e.g., Fontes et al., 2001).

It is far beyond the scope of this chapter to examine sexual abuse prevention strategies in general (see Daro, 1994). (The recently formed Association for Sexual Abuse Prevention [ASAP] has created a virtual online community for sharing resources and experiences in this regard.) Rather, I would like to offer some preliminary reflections on cultural competency in sexual abuse prevention.

Most child sexual abuse prevention programs occur in schools. A 1990 survey of 440 randomly selected elementary school districts in the United States found that 85% offered some such instruction, and 64% mandated its instruction (Finkelhor, Asdigian, & Dzuba-Leatherman, 1993). The best school-based programs usually occur over an extended period of time and involve parents and school personnel as well as children. These programs help children learn to recognize, resist, and tell a trusted adult about uncomfortable situations, from bullying to harassment to "uncomfortable touches" to sexual abuse.

Comprehensive school-based programs have been found to be effective in improving children's knowledge of sexual victimization, increasing children's likelihood of employing self-protection strategies when threatened, and increasing the likelihood that children will disclose victimizations or attempted victimizations (Finkelhor et al., 1993). One recent study examined the possibility that such programs would actually *prevent* abuse. Gibson and Leitenberg (2000) studied 825 women at a state university and found that those who had participated in a child education prevention program were significantly less likely to experience sexual abuse later. The Gibson and Leitenberg study participants were overwhelmingly White.[2] Plummer (2001) notes that 17% of the 87 school-based programs that responded to her survey reported some culturally specific components

---

[2] I have found no information on whether these prevention programs work well with members of immigrant and minority cultural groups.

in their programs. However, she reports no information on the nature of these components. In their facilitator's guide and curriculum on school-based sexual abuse prevention, *Keeping Kids Safe*, Tobin and Kessner (2002) include a section on "respecting differences" that recommends translating materials for monolingual children, using culturally relevant names and scenarios in skits, and using diverse personnel to implement the program. Their drawings, posters, and puppets are either of animals, who evidence no particular cultural or racial characteristics, or of children from a variety of ethnic groups. Their activities are either generic or open enough so children can adapt them to their own situations. These approaches provide a useful starting point for making sure that school-based programs are relevant for all children.

The trademarked Good Touch/Bad Touch program relies on classroom facilitators from children's own communities, including school personnel, social workers, children's advocacy center staff, and police. The program's founder, Pam Church, believes that this makes the program more responsive to children's local and cultural needs (personal communication, August 19, 2003). The curriculum allows children to discuss their own particular concerns, which are sometimes incorporated into new revisions of the curriculum. Church describes some of the issues that have arisen within specific communities:

> In Atlanta's public schools, with low-income African American urban children, food can be a big issue. For example, in one third-grade class children brought up the fact that some children were stealing food from other children in order to eat. No teacher was aware of this problem. Another issue is fear of telling about anything that may involve police. These children have often experienced police coming into their families and taking away children or adults. In rural African American communities in Georgia, children are often poor. An educator wanted us to emphasize with his children that they should not be placed in a position where they must trade their bodies for money. He believed some adults saw the children as "sexually active" because "that is what they do in this culture," which was, of course, incorrect. These young people were being coerced into sexual activity by older men with money.

Church reports that when working in Jewish day schools, she will integrate concepts from the Torah.

These child assault prevention programs in schools would appear to offer great potential to help children stand up for themselves in a variety of areas, including sexual abuse. It would appear that the success of these programs can be aided by a good fit with the children's ethnic culture and socioeconomic circumstances. I look forward to the day when there will be greater research information available about how to achieve this cultural fit between children and programs.

## Culture-Specific Programs

There are two ways for programs to be culturally competent. Some can be culturally *open* and meant to reach *diverse* groups—for example, a public service announcement that is delivered in a way that addresses the needs of various ethnic communities (multicultural), or a school-based program that uses examples relevant to a variety of cultures, as discussed above. Other programs can be targeted to the needs of specific ethnic groups (culture-specific). For instance, a public service announcement on a Spanish language television station is likely to be culture-specific and targeted to Latino viewers. In this section, I discuss agencies and programs geared to preventing child maltreatment within specific communities. This discussion is meant to be suggestive, not comprehensive. Indeed, the lack of a large body to coordinate diverse prevention efforts across states and nations makes it quite difficult to figure out what is being done where. This lack inhibits agencies from pooling their resources and increases the likelihood that organizations will find themselves "reinventing the wheel."

Professionals who work in ethnic communities stress the need to build relationships. "Relationships between individuals may hold more weight than credentials. It is therefore important to take time to build relationships within a community," writes Kelly Ramsden, who works with Aboriginal communities in Australia (personal communication, August 2003). In describing some of the differences in implementing prevention efforts with Aboriginal families in Australia as compared to their efforts in the mainstream, Ramsden writes that they follow "Aboriginal protocols" which vary by community, but generally include:

- Waiting to be invited into a community.
- Allowing the community to set its own agenda and priorities.
- Speaking with tribal elders before initiating a program.
- Allowing more time for each activity so there can be more room for discussions.
- Becoming aware of any community divides or factions and handling these political issues with care.
- Taking community events (e.g., funerals, holidays) into account and understanding that these hold precedence over trainings.
- Finding out about community norms around talking to people of the opposite sex, or kin such as grandparents, about sexual matters, and following these norms.
- Knowing that a professional's own personal commitment will be more highly regarded than the limitations of the organization, and therefore the individual may be expected to bend over backward to be helpful.

- Balancing the above with a professional attitude.
- Forming appropriate same-sex relationships (e.g., with friends, mentors) within the community that gives the professional a "place" within the community.
- Addressing some of the fears that Aboriginal people may have regarding government intervention, caused by past policies encouraging the removal of children from Aboriginal families.

These suggestions are applicable to other groups too, illustrating the kind of care that must be taken by any agency wishing to implement child abuse prevention in a given ethnic community.

It is crucial to partner with community leaders and agencies that are already trusted by their ethnic communities, and to build efforts that make true sense within the ethnic context. These local agencies and leaders are more apt to know the needs and habits of the community than an agency "from outside."

Recently, a number of organizations of various sizes have formed to address child abuse within specific ethnic communities in the United States and Canada. Moreover, some of the larger child abuse prevention organizations have begun adapting their programs to the needs of specific communities. The National Indian Child Welfare Association (NICWA), for instance, offers a positive native parenting course geared to improving the parenting of all native parents.

## Naturalistic Prevention Strategies

Most communities and families engage in what I call "naturalistic" prevention strategies, that is, the things people do (without instruction) to keep their children safe. These efforts can be more or less successful, depending on the child's vulnerability and the degree of threat faced. For example, in the STOP IT NOW! Philadelphia study discussed earlier, we found that African American women described protecting their own children and their nieces, nephews, and grandchildren by telling them to avoid certain people and places, and by caring for their grandchildren and other young relatives themselves, rather than allowing them to be cared for by strangers. Similarly, some Latino men described telling the mothers of their children not to send the children to daycare "with strangers." Some Latinos and African Americans described protecting their daughters from sexual assault by monitoring their clothing and the way they danced, to make sure they would not appear overly seductive or older than their age.

Communities also engage in naturalistic prevention against physical abuse, helping out parents who seem stressed, aiding in the care of developmentally delayed children to support the parents (Maiter, 2003), scolding relatives who are behaving too harshly with their children, and so on. When I was a young mother of a toddler, I remember when once my toddler crumpled a photograph and I shouted at her. My father turned to me and said, "That tone of voice is too harsh for what your daughter did. You need to reserve that for worse infractions!" Although I did not think of it in this way at the time, it is clear that he was intervening as a concerned grandfather to lower the level of parent–child conflict. This was a naturalistic child protection strategy.

To design prevention strategies for specific communities, it might be advisable to assess the naturalistic prevention approaches that currently exist, and then to lend support to enhance these, rather than "importing" strategies that may seem foreign and may be ill-suited to a given community. For example, if parents in a neighborhood or apartment building take turns caring for each other's children, perhaps this process might be enhanced by formal training or organization. Or if young parents turn to the elderly female residents of an apartment building for advice and support, perhaps some of these elderly women could be trained in a way that would enhance their knowledge base and supportive function (see Mosby et al., 1999). Designing prevention programs that build upon naturalistic prevention strategies requires an intimate knowledge of the community. Ideally, prevention professionals would offer leaders from ethnic communities "flexible, empirically based criteria for building their own prevention programs" (Daro & Cohn Donnelly, 2002, p. 440).

## THE PARENTS' BEST INTERESTS

"The best interest of each child is linked to the parents' best interests" (Marneffe, 1996, p. 381). Sometimes we forget this basic truth. When we see children who have been hurt, and we think about the parents who have hurt them or who have failed to protect them, it is easy to view parents mistakenly as the enemy. Marneffe urges us to shift our focus:

> Should we not be more conscious of the fact that the lack of social solidarity at all levels—health care, education, social welfare—in our western societies is the enemy rather than abusive parents, pedophiles, perpetrators, drug addicts, teenage parents, and others. . . . In absence of a public welfare system, it is understandable that reporting systems are implemented to give the community the impression that the State is taking care of the child. . . . Once labeled "child abusers" most families do not receive services except for investigations. (p. 380)

If we broaden our lens to see the big picture, then we approach prevention at a different level: that of the society rather than of the individual.

Epidemiologists assert that there are two ways to prevent disease: preventing individual cases or lowering the incidence in a given population (Rose, 1992). We can incorporate this concept into our thinking about preventing child maltreatment. Understanding why an individual case of maltreatment occurs is not necessarily the same as understanding why maltreatment might occur with greater frequency in a given population. Child maltreatment prevention professionals work almost exclusively at the individual level. That is, education, sanctions, or support are provided to individual caretakers to help them stop engaging in private acts of maltreatment or neglect. These efforts range from public service announcements (e.g., "Don't shake your baby!") to home visitation to psychotherapy. Each of these approaches shares an attempt to intervene on the level of the "case" or family, and each is important.

A prevention method based on incidence would ask why there are higher levels of maltreatment among certain populations—for example, more physical abuse and child neglect among people who have low incomes, are unemployed, who abuse drugs, or who live in deteriorated neighborhoods. To lower the incidence in this population, professionals could either target this population with prevention services (again, the individualistic approach, but this time targeted to a specific population) or attempt to address the root causes of this increased incidence. The association between extremely low income and physical abuse has proved to be robust over time. The most effective way to reduce abuse among those at the bottom of the social ladder may well be to provide jobs, quality housing, and income subsidies, thereby addressing the stresses of poverty, rather than simply offering home visitation and/or parenting classes. Addressing societal injustice, rather than presumed parental deficiencies, requires greater commitment. It requires us to admit that if some of us were forced to live in the circumstances in which some of our clients live, we too might hurt our children, and certainly might be unable to provide for them adequately.

## ADDRESSING PHYSICAL ABUSE: PARENT GROUPS AND CLASSES

This section is intended to help professionals address parenting problems in a group setting in culturally respectful ways. While running abuse prevention groups and classes for parents, facilitators often wonder how to work well with parents from different cultural backgrounds. Specifically, they may puzzle over how to engage with parents from diverse groups, how to help parents draw the line between discipline and abuse in a culturally respectful way, how to respect various communication styles while promoting a reduction in family conflict, how to create a supportive environment for people from varying backgrounds who participate in the group together, and how to reduce mistrust of the child welfare system and other government agencies.

This query below, posted on a list-serve for professionals who work in child maltreatment, describes some of the difficulties:

> I'm giving a workshop this Friday on child discipline, something I've taught about many times. This time, though, the audience is a group of family support workers. They are mostly African American, as are their clients; in addition, many are conservative Christians raised on the "spare the rod" lore. Many believe that spanking is an acceptable form of discipline. . . . I've just learned that this argument [about spanking] has torpedoed previous trainings with this group on this subject, as workers demand to know if the speaker has ever spanked a child, why they can't teach parents about spanking, and that the speaker does not understand the rigors of raising a compliant child in a terrible environment.

List-serve respondents offered a variety of suggestions about how to address issues of child discipline and physical abuse in groups involving a culture that is different from the trainer's, including the best teacher/worst boss exercise (discussed below), asking parents to recall what it felt like to be punished as a child, and asking parents to describe a time someone they know "went too far" in punishing a child.

Over a decade ago when I did my first workshop for the Georgia Council on Child Abuse (now Prevent Child Abuse Georgia), I watched as my training session on child maltreatment sank fast because of my own cultural ignorance. There were about 150 participants in the workshop including about 120 African American front-line protective workers and parent aides. When I brought up the issue of discipline there was practically a civil war in the room. I sat in awe and watched for a while because people were so impassioned. Luckily, not all the anger was addressed at me. There were two opposing opinions, both stated firmly and clearly. One group argued that corporal punishment was a key element of African American parenting, and any attempt to challenge it was a form of cultural domination bordering on genocide. And the other group argued that the practice of physical discipline was a form of self-hate or internalized oppression among African Americans, perhaps even a relic of slavery, and must be eliminated. A handful of people who held the first opinion were so incensed by those who held the second that they simply walked out of the workshop in disgust.

Since that time, I have run several other successful workshops on the same topic for the same audience in Georgia and elsewhere—but now I come prepared with strategies and tips to help prevent these groups from self-destructing. (I discuss these below.) I have found ways to introduce this sensitive discussion that allow people to open their minds rather than immediately become defensive.

This anecdote illustrates several important points: that diversity exists even among people of similar cultural backgrounds, that group facilitators must create the kind of environment where diverse opinions can be expressed, and that facilitators should become familiar with the norms of the cultural group with whom they'll be working to avoid unpleasant and sometimes volatile surprises.

## Marketing Parenting Groups or Classes in Diverse Communities

Some parents resent the suggestion or mandate that they attend a parenting *class*. Indeed, these referrals are often inappropriate. Parents who live fairly stable lives and want the best for their children but lack parenting skills can benefit from parenting classes. Parents who actively dislike a certain child, who are intentionally cruel and malicious to that child, or who are overwhelmed by their own psychopathology, substance abuse, or life circumstances may need other interventions first. A mother who is in a battering relationship is *not* a good candidate for a parenting class—she may risk her life if she opposes her violent partner's behaviors, and her partner may use abuse against the child as another way to control her (Bancroft & Silverman, 2002).

Parenting classes may not be the best referral if the parent has severe mental health challenges, or is an active abuser of substances, or had parented well until a recent stressor (e.g., homelessness). The parent may need help first with mental health issues, treatment for substance abuse, or assistance with a concrete problem (such as housing) rather than instructions in how to parent. Some parents like the idea of attending a *class* or a *discussion group* more than they like the idea of attending a *therapy group* because a group implies the sharing of one's private concerns and it sounds like psychotherapy. Culturally, many members of ethnic minority groups think therapy is only for people who are *crazy*, and they may especially resist the idea of airing their dirty laundry in public in a group setting. Group facilitators and planners should think carefully about how to market the parenting group or class to the particular population in a nonpathologizing way.

For instance, a group called "Teen Years Are Tough: Learn What Works" is apt to be more appealing than "Support Group for Abusive Parents of Teenagers." Similarly, Chinese immigrant parents might be more receptive to attending a class called "Parenting Children in the United States" than they would be to a parenting class in general. Attending the first implies that they need to learn tips for handling children in their new culture, whereas the second implies remediating a deficit in their general parenting abilities.

In practice, groups and classes are often mixed. One group I co-facilitated began with a 10-minute didactic piece on child development at the opening of each session—describing what to expect at a certain age—and then allowed people to discuss whatever had come up for them with their children that week. This combination of new information with mutual support seemed to appeal to parents. To obtain insurance reimbursement we needed to describe the gathering as a psychotherapy group, which it was—but we avoided using this phrase in our conversations with parents.

## Group or Class Composition

Should parenting groups or classes be homogeneous or heterogeneous? This question is more complicated than it may first appear. Which aspects are we considering: Race? Social class? Being an immigrant or not? A recent immigrant from El Salvador may have more in common with a recent immigrant from Albania than he would with a Latino who has been in the United States for five generations. And upper-middle-class African American parents may share more of the same concerns with White upper-middle-class parents than they do with low-income African American parents.

Some parents prefer to be in a group with parents like themselves. Others prefer a mixed group. By all means, if you have enough people who would rather do a parenting group in Spanish, then put them together. You may not have a choice about the composition of your group. If at all possible, avoid a situation where a parent or a couple is the only one from their ethnicity, social class, or sexual orientation—or at least warn them that this might be happening and ask if that's acceptable to them. If not, perhaps they could help recruit more participants from their own background, or they might be willing to accept a referral to another group with parents who are more similar to them. If a parent or a couple is the only one from their identity group in a parenting class (e.g., the only Black or lesbian couple), it will be hard for them to speak freely about their struggles—they may experience the pressure of having to represent their identity group favorably. This is an unfair burden.

A skilled facilitator can handle a group with diverse backgrounds and perspectives. The facilitator needs to create an open atmosphere so that people can learn from one another:

"Hey, we're a mixed group of parents here. We probably have a lot of different ideas in this room. I'm not expecting us all to agree on every-thing. It is important to respect each other and each other's ideas. Rich or poor, Black or White, male or female, every parent has a hard time sometimes, and every parent has ideas that would be helpful to oth-ers."

When at all possible, parents should be able to attend groups where they can speak in their native language. Having an interpreter means that the non-English-speaking member is on an unequal footing with the other members; this should be avoided.

## Group Leadership Style

Do not just "talk at" parents in the didactic portion of your group or class, if you have one. Involvement increases memory. If you can tell a story that moves people emotionally, they are more likely to remember it. If you can design an activity that illustrates a point, or allows your participants to in-teract or practice a technique, this is even better. The more you say, the less they'll remember. Keep it simple.

More experienced facilitators are usually comfortable being "a guide from the side rather than a sage from the stage," at least some of the time. This may vary with the length of the group and its goals. Many facilitators try to use some activities where they are central, and others where the par-ticipants interact with each other with little facilitator input, in pairs or as a group.

Many experienced group leaders have participants set the norms at the beginning of the first session, and then post them on the wall for later sessions. If the participants set the rules—such as no interrupting, don't hog the floor, respect others' opinions, and so on—the parents are apt to help you enforce those norms. And you can always point back to the list es-tablished by the group.

If you are in the unfortunate situation of being from a more dominant social group than that of your clients—let's say you are a White person working with Latino participants, or an upper-middle-class African Amer-ican working with lower income participants—it will be especially impor-tant for you to share the power and let people know that *you know* that *they know* a lot. In this situation, I strongly recommend recruiting a likeminded co-facilitator who is closer in background to the group participants.

I think it's easier for parents to bond with the facilitators if at least one of the facilitators is from the same cultural group. Let me tell you how I might handle this if I were asked to lead a parenting group for Latino parents. First, I'd try to get a co-facilitator who was Latino whom I liked to work with. If that failed, I would introduce myself in a way that identified what I know and what I have in common with the participants, and what I don't know. I might say the following:

> "I am not Latina. You may wonder why I'm being asked to lead this class today. Let's look at what we have in common. We are all parents. I have three kids of my own. I live in an immigrant family. Not only are my own grandparents immigrants, but my husband is an immigrant too who didn't speak English when I met him. I've been speaking Spanish since I was 17. I have many Latino friends, and I am committed, heart and soul, to making the social service system work better for Latinos. But I do *not* know what it is to be in your shoes, and you've had many experiences that I have not had. So while I'm teaching you some things about child development, and I'll be teaching you some things about how the social service system works in this country, I expect you'll be teaching me a lot too about your own ideas and families and cultures. *Cuando meto la pata* [when I put my foot in my mouth] I'm counting on you to let me know. Any questions?"

Again, I do advocate for at least one of the two group leaders to be from the same ethnic group as the participants. However, a brief introduction like the one above has worked for me when co-facilitation was not possible.

## Co-facilitation

Co-facilitating a group can be wonderful. You can demonstrate how to coparent and do role plays. You can demonstrate how to disagree respectfully. You can present a variety of viewpoints. You have someone to plan with and discuss what happened in the group, and you can supervise each other, learn from each other, and support each other. One of you can take the lead while the other sits back, and there's someone to cover if one facilitator is absent. Ideally, co-facilitators should each bring an area of diversity: a man and a woman, a White and a Black, an older person and a younger person, and so on. But if the chemistry isn't right, co-facilitating a group can be almost as trying as coparenting with an ill-suited partner. Decisions about co-facilitation should be made carefully. And co-facilitation should not take the place of supervision.

## Handouts

Handouts give people something to take home, think about, discuss with their families, and refer to between group sessions. They reinforce learning. The form these handouts take might vary with the culture of the participants. For instance, child abuse prevention messages written on a bookmark are not apt to be useful with a group of parents who are only marginally literate. However, simple phrases or drawings on a piece of paper that can be hung on the refrigerator or cartoon representations of the day's lesson can serve as a useful reminder and topic of discussion for participants to bring home. Some facilitators ask participants to draw up their own reminders.

Other options include giving people a small card with helpful information or reminders. Religious individuals may decide to place these in their Bibles; others will place them in their wallets or purses, in their pockets, or on their car dashboards. Some facilitators will ask each person at the end of a session to think of a lesson he or she would like to remember from the group or class, and then write it on a small card to carry with them. Alternatively, facilitators can give each participant a small stone or bead and encourage participants to carry it with them during the week, and rub it when they want to remember the lessons of the group.

## Discussing Controversial Issues

It may be important to address issues of culture, discrimination, and racism where relevant. For instance, if I'm working with a group that is of a different ethnicity than mine, I might say, "You know, some Latinos say that most children in this country are too wild and disrespectful. Do you agree?" After hearing the group's response, which might take a while to emerge, I might say:

> "In this group I am not here to impose on you anyone's ideas of what your kids should be like. If you want your kids to listen, I'd like to help you do that. If you believe strongly in the value of respect, I'd like to help you get more respect from your children. But I'd like to help you to do it in ways that are not violent, and won't get you into trouble."

It may be important to acknowledge that the contexts in which diverse parents raise children are not the same. African American parents, in particular, often report that they need to raise their children—and especially their boys—to behave properly in a hostile world. The fear of police assault and brutality is palpable in some African American communities, and it drives some parents to try to beat their sons into obedience. Where this is the case, it would be important for facilitators to recognize, aloud, the fear of police brutality and the ways this fear can affect parenting. Low-income parents may be reassured by hearing a professional empathize with how difficult it is to raise children with the stressors of economic uncertainty, difficult housing, poor schools, discrimination, and so on. The professional must be sure to convey an attitude of genuine empathy and solidarity, not condescension or paternalism.

## Ways to Begin the Group: Setting the Tone

Some of the issues of setting the right tone were discussed earlier, in terms of what the group is called, how and where it is advertised, and who facilitates it. The physical setting for the group is also important. The meeting room should have sufficient space and flexible seating so people can break into small groups. Extra chairs should be removed. The room should be as clean and pleasant as possible. We communicate that group members are valuable by meeting with them in a pleasant environment. And the meeting space should be private and nonpathologizing. For example, a group held in a school, church basement, YMCA, or other community center is apt to seem less problematic than a group held in the building of the state society on the abuse of children—even if the content and the facilitators are identical.

## Some Other Tips

• Give parents an opportunity to introduce themselves in a positive light. Ask, for example, "What do you do best as a parent?" or "What is your favorite thing about being a parent?"

• Acknowledge the difficulty of being a parent and the impossibility of being a perfect parent. Tell stories that acknowledge your own imperfections.

• Be warm, accepting, and friendly. Acknowledge each person by name and try to connect with each person around a specific detail in his or her life (e.g., to a mother as she enters the group room, "How is Johnny's toothache this week, Ms. Morales?"). Many people lack this kind of acknowledgment and this sense of being known, particularly if they have recently moved into the area. This connection with the facilitator can give participants impetus to return each week.

• Give participants an opportunity to laugh with each other and at themselves. For example, you can share funny stories from your own experience as a parent, or ask parents to write down cute or funny experiences they have with their children and share them each week.

• Some programs have used innovative incentives to increase parental participation, engagement, and retention. One program provided stress-reducing acupuncture to caretakers who attended after the fourth week, introducing the acupuncture as an additional way to reduce stress

(U.S. Department of Health and Human Services, Administration for Children and Families, 2003).

• Do activities where participants practice behaviors related to the materials you've discussed that week. Have parents commit to trying out a specific technique each week and then report back to the group on the success of their attempts. Make sure that these are occasions for mutual support and encouragement, not shaming.

• Be clear about the limits on confidentiality in the screening or orientation to the group or class. For example, if you will be reporting to the courts or child protective services that a parent attended X number of sessions, the parent should know this. At the same time, if you will *not* be reporting the content of what a parent says, except for the obvious exception of a new disclosure of child abuse, the parent should know this as well. Some parents will be unnecessarily concerned that everything they say or do in a parenting group will be reported back to their caseworkers.

• Give parents an opportunity to connect with each other. The parenting groups give caretakers an opportunity to reduce their isolation and to build relationships that may extend over time. Activities may be conducted in pairs or in small groups. People should be told to avoid pairing with their coparents for certain activities. In certain cultural groups, such as some Muslims, Amish, and Orthodox Jews, these groups should be same-sex rather than cross-sex. Providing snacks can allow for easier bonding, and may improve attendance and retention.

## Discussing Discipline in Parenting Groups

Chapter 5 provides useful ideas for facilitators of parent groups on this subject. The following are tips for group activities:

• Facilitators can have parents brainstorm a list of discipline techniques that are *not* good or that they think are too harsh. You can start off with something they all agree on—such as that hitting a child over the head with a hammer is too dangerous. But beyond this, there may be great disagreement. This discussion will enable parents to see others struggling with similar issues. If facilitated well, it can also help parents become aware of some of the factors that need to be considered when thinking about discipline issues including the child's age, health, and stress level; the infraction; previous warnings; and so on.

• Some facilitators ask participants to share a memory of a time when they themselves were punished as a child, describing what happened, how they felt then, and how they feel about it now. (Some parents will decline to participate in this exercise—they will feel that it is too intimate.) During this discussion, parents frequently laugh or smile as they discuss painful or humiliating experiences. I like to point this out and ask the group why people so often laugh when discussing childhood experiences of being punished. Participants usually say things like "I'm embarrassed" or "I feel like a naughty child again." This discussion usually increases the level of intimacy in the group, and helps participants avoid some of the minimizing that frequently occurs. Additionally, when participants cut quickly from "At the time I felt embarrassed and humiliated" to "But now I appreciate what my parents did for me," I encourage them to remain with the child's experience for a while, before moving into the adult's evaluation of that experience. Recalling the *child's* experience of punishment can help parents empathize more closely with their own children.

• Have parents use crayons to draw on a piece of paper something that has to do with a time when they were punished physically as a child. After a few minutes, have each person describe his or her drawing.

• Have parents brainstorm a list of problems with using corporal punishment (e.g., it can become abusive, it can look abusive to others, it's tiring, it doesn't work after a certain age, sometimes children get hurt, sometimes parents feel bad afterward). Engage parents in a discussion of these problems. Consider hanging the list on the wall, or typing it up and distributing it.

## One Final Caution: Honor Participants' Parents

Nothing sabotages a group more quickly than giving participants the impression that you are insulting their own parents. This can be particularly true when working with parents from cultures that highly value respecting elders, such as African Americans, Latinos, and Asian Americans. I recommend that during the introduction of a group the facilitator say something of this kind:

> "By the last session of this group, I expect you'll change your mind, at least a little, about some of the ways you handle your children. You'll probably continue doing a lot of the things that you're doing now, because they are working; and you'll probably also decide to try some new behaviors. You may decide that some of the ways your parents raised you are not the ways you want to raise your own children. Now, before we get any further, let me say that I am *not* saying anything bad about anyone's mama. Our parents did the best they knew how. But times have changed, and what we do as parents has to change with the times. Many parents who are loving and very skilled still use certain parenting techniques that cause more harm than good. I recognize that this approach can bring up loyalty issues for some people. 'If I decide to do something different from what my parents

did, am I being disloyal to them, or rejecting them, or saying they weren't good parents?' No. You can decide to give up *some* of the ways your parents treated you, and still preserve the values they gave you that you like. Did any of you, when you were growing up, ever have a dish served to you that you hated? In my family it was corned beef. Now I love my parents, and I do a lot of things that my parents did, but I will *not* serve my children corned beef. You may find that there are certain practices—just like certain dishes—that were served up in your family growing up that you're ready to abandon, even as you keep and treasure others."

The good news about parenting groups and classes is that they seem to work, if they are run well. Daro and Cohn Donnelly (2001) write that parents who have participated in center-based parenting education and services demonstrate gains in parenting skills and the use of community resources, including

> an increase in positive parent–child interactions, more extensive use of social supports, less use of corporal punishment, and higher self-esteem and personal functioning. For teen mothers, positive outcomes also include fewer subsequent births, higher employment rates, and less welfare dependency. (p. 437)

It may be obvious, but it is still worth stating, that these groups will only succeed if the caretakers attend them. This requires scheduling that is sensitive to caretakers' needs, geographic proximity to where potential clients live, provision of transportation, and free onsite childcare, whenever possible. If facilitators are able to provide a beverage and snack, this will stave off absenteeism and boost group morale, particularly for those parents for whom food resources may get stretched thin each month.

## CONCLUDING THOUGHTS

Ultimately, preventing child abuse and neglect is the key to keeping all children safe. Prevention efforts need to reach all children and families, and particularly those who are at added risk because they live in precarious economic circumstances. A first step to reducing child abuse and neglect certainly includes securing steady food, housing, and education for all children and employment for adults.

To be successful, prevention efforts should reach all levels of a child's ecosystem: the child him- or herself, home and family, ethnic culture, proximal systems such as schools and neighborhood, and the nation. Professionals must create relationships and true partnerships with leaders and families from culturally diverse communities. This requires culturally competent communications, prevention services that are easily accessed by people from those communities, and parenting groups that "make sense" within the client's cultural worldview.

## QUESTIONS TO THINK ABOUT AND DISCUSS

1. Describe some of the particular challenges for child maltreatment prevention programs in serving the diverse people in your area.

2. Design a child maltreatment prevention approach to reach members of a population described in the first question.

3. In what ways do you think your own identity (e.g., race, gender, ethnicity, religion, age, etc.) affects your ability to conduct parenting groups with members of diverse cultures in your area?

4. How would you approach an immigrant family that had acted in a physically abusive way toward a child, but that had not been aware of the laws and expectations in their new country?

# CHAPTER NINE

# Improving the Cultural Competency of Your Child Maltreatment Agency or Organization

I hope you have acquired helpful ideas for improving the cultural competency of your work in child maltreatment through reading this book. This chapter focuses on the changes that need to be made on the level of agencies and organizations to improve our ability to serve culturally diverse people impacted by child maltreatment. While this chapter may be most immediately relevant to supervisors, administrators, policymakers, and people who aspire to those positions, I hope others will read it too. Often agency and community changes happen through the hard work of people on the front lines who make their voices heard—instituting change from the bottom up.

An individual professional can become well versed in the needs of culturally diverse clients, familiar with his or her own cultural background and biases, and engaged in a process of achieving cultural competency. But if the climate in which that person works is *not* supportive of staff and clients from diverse backgrounds, and if that agency's policies are discriminatory, there are limits to what even the best-intentioned individual can do. Just as individuals develop and improve, agencies do, too. An agency that is engaged in a process of achieving cultural competency is more than just a collection of individuals who are doing the same. Ideally, the agency has conducted an assessment, set clear goals, set timelines for achieving those goals, and assigned tasks that will bring the agency closer to those goals. This process should be repeated every few years. Ideally, linguistic and cultural competence goals should be incorporated into all strategic planning, and related measures should be incorporated into all evaluations, self-assessments, and client satisfaction surveys (U.S. Department of Health and Human Services, 2001).

A number of useful models have been developed for understanding multicultural organizational development, with a variety of stages outlined. Here I briefly describe Sue and Sue's (2003) three-stage model. At one end of the spectrum are *monocultural organizations*, which are primarily Eurocentric and ethnocentric and which do not take cultural diversity into account. In these agencies, the clients and staff at all levels are encouraged to assimilate. In the middle of the spectrum are *nondiscriminatory organizations*, which have inconsistent policies and practices regarding multicultural issues. While some agency professionals may become sensitive to minority issues, the agency itself lacks a systemic policy to address prejudice and bias. Changes that are implemented to promote diversity may be superficial. At the other end of the spectrum are *multicultural organizations* that see diversity as an asset; this commitment is infused throughout the organization. They are continually engaged in visioning, planning, and problem-solving activities to allow for equal access and opportunities, and to improve their ability to address the needs of diverse professionals and clients. You might want to think about where on the spectrum your agency falls, and how you can push it forward to achieve greater multicultural competence.

## WHY SHOULD AGENCIES CHANGE?

In the sections below, I provide examples of less-than-adequate agency practices, followed by a discussion of the changes that would make a difference.

### Improving Sensitivity and Providing Orientation to the Process

Calvin, a 20-year-old African American college student, was skeptical about going for counseling, but his basketball coach recommended it when Calvin confessed one day that he occasionally suffered from angry outbursts and crying spells, and indicated that he had had some "bad stuff" happen to him in his childhood. Calvin made an appointment at his local counseling center, where he submitted to an intake interview with a 40-year-old White woman, Betsy. Using her considerable empathic skills, Betsy was able to coax Calvin into describing childhood sexual abuse and his witnessing of domestic violence. Toward the end of the interview Betsy explained that she would not be his counselor, but rather was going to talk about his "case" to the team, who would then decide together who would be the best psychotherapist for him. Calvin grew angry, told Betsy that she shouldn't have gotten him to open up if she didn't want to work with him, demanded his paperwork and her notes, ripped them up, and walked out.

Several issues become evident here. First, that particular agency was set up in a way that requires the client to discuss his or her issues with at least two people: the intake coordinator and then the therapist. While this may be comfortable or even routine for someone from a culture that values the open sharing of problems, it might be experienced as unnecessary and unproductive for a client like Calvin, who may be mistrustful of therapy and therapists from the beginning. If the agency hopes to work well with a person like Calvin, it might want to think about altering its intake process to minimize the necessity of self-revelation to more than one person. Or at the very least it should explain the process carefully from the beginning of the intake meeting, perhaps even cautioning the client that he or she does not need to reveal too much at this first meeting, and letting him or her know the reasons why the person conducting the intake is not the same person who provides the psychotherapy.

The agency described above appears to have a set routine way of working with clients, and seems to expect the clients to conform to this practice. The process may feel alien and alienating for people who are less familiar with the psychotherapeutic world. Ideally, such an agency would reexamine its intake process and ask itself whether it is the best process for all clients, or how it can be improved so that it supports—rather than scares away—a client like Calvin.

## Altering Agency Decor

A Lebanese family was contacted when their daughter's third-grade teacher was found to have sexually fondled another child in the class. The parents brought their daughter in for an interview at the local children's advocacy center to determine if she too had been abused. They were predisposed to cooperate until they entered the center and saw a big American flag hanging in the lobby and patriotic banners decorating the waiting room. The parents suddenly felt uncomfortable. They met with the interviewer and told her that they had changed their minds and would not allow their daughter to be interviewed.

Achieving cultural competency is never as simple as hanging an "ethnic" wall-hanging in the waiting room. On the other hand, people from diverse groups should be able to feel welcomed and at home as they walk into our agencies; the decor can help set the tone. Books, magazines, artwork, signs, photographs, and posters in all the rooms and hallways should reflect the variety of cultures served. People from minority ethnic and racial groups will frequently scan their environment for visible signs that the agency recognizes their existence and needs (e.g., Are the signs in Spanish as well as English? Are a variety of holidays represented in the decorations, or only Christian holidays such as Christmas? Is there a copy of *Essence* magazine next to the copy of the *Ladies' Home Journal*?). Invite members of the local community to have a say in the decoration of your agency facility. This is apt to increase feelings of connection to the agency as well as make the decor more interesting and culturally welcoming.

Some agencies in Latino neighborhoods allow their clients to set up altars on agency premises. The clients adorn the altars with photographs, personal possessions, flowers, and other small offerings, much as they would do in the small Central American villages where many of them once lived. The agencies recognize their clients' cultures in this way, and give them a safe space to practice it without imposing it on clients from other groups. The opportunity to face an altar, collect their thoughts, and compose themselves before and after sessions related to sexual trauma or domestic violence serves as a bridge for the clients between their old world and the new, and between the safe psychotherapeutic space and the rest of the world. Some domestic violence support groups use these altars to honor other women who suffered or died at the hands of their intimate partners (Gloria de la Cruz Quiroz, personal communication, 2004).

Flags and patriotic slogans and symbols adorn many waiting rooms and buildings in the United States since the September 11, 2001, terrorist attacks. Some people feel their desire to express their patriotic sentiments quite strongly. They may have trouble understanding how off-putting these nationalistic symbols can be to people from other nations. This was driven home to me when I conducted a week-long training for Spanish-speaking interviewers in a conference room with an enormous U.S. flag hanging on the wall. The participants from El Salvador and Nicaragua let me know that awful things had been done in their country in the name of that flag. Upon my request, a staff member removed the flag for the next day's sessions. On the third morning, an administrator informed me that some employees were upset that the flag had been taken down, and the administrator insisted on hanging it up again. Clearly, this issue is a passionate one for many people. My recommendation is that we err on the side of being as welcoming and inclusive to as many people as possible in our professional lives. Therefore, I believe that patriotic and political symbols are not appropriate in most workplaces, particularly those that serve immigrant and undocumented clients. As with the Lebanese family described above, we may never know how many people decide not to seek our services, refuse our services, limit what they say, or decline to cooperate because they do not feel at ease in our agencies. We should do whatever we can to extend the welcome to all potential clients.

## Supporting Bilingual Professionals and Providing Quality Services for Everyone

> Child protective services in a city with growing immigrant populations has decided to hire its first Spanish- and Vietnamese-speaking social workers. Elena and Boret are hired fresh out of college, and within 6 months they have the largest caseloads in the agency. All families who do not speak English or who are of Latino or Asian background are automatically referred to them. In addition, they are often interrupted during their workday to interpret for their colleagues. Two years down the road, they have both left the agency. Their supervisor and colleagues wonder why they "just couldn't take it," and are hesitant to hire bilingual/bicultural professionals in the future. What happened, and how can an agency work to hire and also retain bilingual and bicultural professionals?

These young professionals were given an impossible task. They were given larger caseloads than their colleagues. In addition, because they were working with immigrant families, it is quite possible that their caseloads were more complex than others'—involving more children per family and greater case coordination responsibilities due to language and cultural differences. As if this wasn't enough, their agencies were expecting them to interpret for their colleagues as a kind of unacknowledged and uncompensated "add-on" to their job.

Bilingual professionals must be protected from these kinds of exploitive conditions. An agency must be fair in its assignment of cases. If there are more cases than the bilingual professional(s) can handle, then additional bilingual staff should be hired, or the monolingual professionals need to engage the services of a professional interpreter—bilingual professionals simply cannot be expected to "absorb" more than their share of cases. If bilingual professionals are going to be expected to serve as interpreters, they should receive training in interpreting, and have their interpreting tasks counted toward their workload (see Chapter 7). They should receive supervision in their native language as well as in English so they can discuss the cultural, linguistic, and systemic issues that may arise with their immigrant clients.

In attempting to address the needs of cultural minority groups, agencies sometimes unwittingly provide separate and unequal services. For example, in my area agencies frequently recruit people with undergraduate degrees in psychology or social work from Puerto Rico to work with Latino clients, whereas English-speaking clients are treated by clinicians with graduate degrees and extensive advanced training. While the agency administrators are well intentioned in trying to fill an urgent need for bilingual professionals, the results are not always as positive as they would have hoped. Language competency alone is not adequate—the professionals also must have clinical knowledge, sophistication, and familiarity with issues of child abuse. Clients from linguistic minority groups are entitled to receive the same quality services as clients from the dominant group, even though such services may be harder to provide.

## Creating a Supportive Work Environment

Brian was the only African American member of the police force in a college town with a small but growing Black population. Every time an African American was arrested or suspected of a crime, the other officers told him "It's one of your cousins" or called in the report with "It's a Brian." When there was an altercation between some Black and White students on campus, one of the officers said, "It's the Brians against the rest of us." Someone hung a picture of a monkey on Brian's locker and taped a picture of a monkey to his coffee mug. After a couple of years Brian left the force and moved to a bigger city with a more racially integrated police force.

The racially hostile environment described above is not only discouraging and difficult for the person who finds himself the target of so much racial attention, but it also constitutes an illegal form of employment discrimination. Racial harassment (like other forms of harassment) is illegal because it interferes with the professional's ability to do his or her job. In this case, not only was Brian's worklife made unpleasant because of his colleagues' comments and actions, but the police force lost an employee who might have been particularly important in reaching the town's growing Black population.

Brian's coworkers might argue that their comments and actions were made without malicious intent, but their intent does not matter much. By constantly referring to Brian's race they let Brian know repeatedly that he was an outsider and was not accepted. The monkey references let him know that someone on the force saw him as less than human. His colleagues and supervisors had a legal and moral obligation to put a stop to the harassment.

## Fostering Integrated Agencies

> Jimmy Clark was adopted at birth from Korea into a White American family in New Hampshire. He is a social worker with child protective services. His supervisor assigns all the Asian American cases to him even though Jimmy has explained several times that he does not speak an Asian language and is more Yankee than Korean.

The staff and board of an agency should reflect the cultural mix of the population in the area. Agencies should recruit, welcome, mentor, support, and retain diverse people at all levels. An agency that is having trouble recruiting diverse staff should examine its hiring priorities. For example, I sometimes speak with directors of children's advocacy centers who report that they are having difficulty recruiting Spanish-speaking bilingual professionals to serve as interviewers and other staff. When I ask to see their job posting, it almost invariably solicits applications from people with a master's degree in social work (MSW) with several years of professional experience in child abuse, and only toward the bottom says, "bilingual/bicultural preferred." While a degree in social work is certainly a fine credential, for many positions an MSW may *not* be necessary—a master's degree in education or counseling may be fine. In fact, there may be people with bachelor's degrees who have experience working with children and families and who could serve in some of the advocacy center positions. By restricting themselves narrowly along professional lines, the centers may be unnecessarily deterring many potential high quality bilingual applicants from applying. However, the pool of bilingual social workers may just be too small in a given area to meet the need. If bilingual or multicultural capabilities are a priority, this should be mentioned early in the ad. Word of mouth can also be an effective recruitment tool. Agencies should send notices about available positions to their contacts within ethnic communities.

Diverse staff including members of all the major cultures in the area is a great advantage, regardless of whether cultural matching between clients and professionals is routinely employed. A diverse treatment team communicates an openness toward culture that may be key to work in minority communities. Diversifying staff to reflect the catchment area has been found to lead to an increased flow of minority clients and increased satisfaction with services (Cooper & Powe, 2004). A diverse team (in terms of training, age, gender, class, religion, race, ethnicity, sexual orientation, and ability) improves an agency's ability to generate creative approaches to diverse client experiences. This hiring needs to be more than a token effort, and the hiring of diverse peoples should be well thought out. An agency needs to think of the problem it is trying to address, and how the new person hired might meet the need. Is it looking for someone with bilingual and bicultural skills? If so, how is it assessing whether the person it is interviewing is truly bilingual and familiar with the cultures of the clients with whom he or she will be working? This assessment must be more thorough than asking the applicant about his or her last name or country of origin.

What kinds of "diversity" matter in terms of hiring? People who are less familiar with a certain group might not be aware of the needs of that group. For instance, in the example cited above, Jimmy was thought to bring diversity to the team because he was originally from Korea, and then all the Asian American cases were assigned to him. However, Jimmy had no special knowledge of Asia, and—in fact—the long-simmering resentment among people of various Asian backgrounds sometimes impeded Jimmy's ability to work with Japanese and Chinese Americans. His Korean clients often resented Jimmy's inability to speak Korean and his lack of familiarity with Korean cultural norms. Jimmy may have been a valuable member of the team for many reasons—including his personal familiarity with the adoption process—but he was not the resource on Asian culture that the agency was seeking. However, a social worker of Mexican background who had served in the Peace Corps in Thailand proved to be a valuable resource for working with Cambodian immigrants who had lived in refugee camps in Thailand. In other words, what matters is not *simply* a question of who people *are*, but also what they *know*, their commitments, and their community participation.

## Democratizing a Diverse Workplace

> Three White male pediatricians in their 40s are looking for a fourth person to join their practice. Although they recognize that hiring a woman or a person from one of the ethnic groups in their area would enhance their ability to treat culturally diverse patients and their families, in the end they decide on another White male of the same age, rationalizing that they need to feel comfortable working with this person, and that having nurses, secretaries, and technicians who are women or from cultural minority groups is "good enough" in terms of their diversity goals.

If the upper levels of an agency are monocultural, the hiring of diverse people at lower levels looks like a form of tokenism, and may deprive the agency of the full benefit of the diverse experience and opinions of the staff. Diverse clients and staff alike perceive who is truly powerful within the organization, and they are less likely to trust an organization with directors, supervisors, and managers who all come from the same cultural group. A similar process can happen in an academic setting. Frequently, research teams consist of White professionals with PhD's who are assisted by a more diverse group of graduate students, who have little voice in the designing of the research. One African American graduate research assistant told me about asking an African American grandmother a question as part of a study that she was helping to implement. A White professor had designed the study questions without asking for her input. The grandmother burst into laughter and said, "Now I *know* you didn't write that question!" In other words, services must be designed and continually evaluated and redesigned with input from members of the community that is served. For an agency to be more than monocultural, it must have diverse staff at all levels of the hierarchy. The Office of Minority Health describes having a diverse staff and leadership that represent the demographic characteristics of an agency's geographic area as a "necessary but not sufficient condition for providing culturally and linguistically appropriate health care services" (U.S. Department of Health and Human Services, 2001, p. 34).

## Paying Attention to Boundaries and Looking for Strengths

Ms. Echeverría was visited one day by a child protective services (CPS) social worker, who told her that her 6-year-old daughter, Carlita, had told her first-grade teacher that Ms. Echeverría's boyfriend, Raúl, had been fondling her sexually. Ms. Echeverría believed her daughter, and demanded that Raúl move out to his mother's house that very night. The CPS social worker visited the family repeatedly over the next few weeks. Ms. Echeverría felt blamed at each visit, and could not understand why she was considered at fault, since she had protected her daughter as soon as she found out about the abuse. The CPS worker insisted that the mother bring Carlita and her siblings to a children's advocacy center for interviews, demanded that the mother take out a restraining order against Raúl, and told Ms. Echeverría that Raúl had ruined the girl's life and that she'd need many years of therapy to recover. The worker told Ms. Echeverría that she'd be visiting unannounced frequently, and that she'd "better not catch Raúl on the premises during one of the visits." One day when the social worker appeared at the door, she saw that the apartment had been emptied. The family had left no forwarding address.

People who have been abused have already had their boundaries violated. Members of oppressed groups also experience violations: they are more likely to have suffered from social service agencies, immigration authorities, and the criminal justice system behaving intrusively with their families. We must be careful not to repeat this victimization. Beyond the obvious injunction against dual relationships, we should try to allow our clients to shape and set the pace of the work together. At each step, we need to ask ourselves and our supervisors, "Am I heading in this particular direction for the client's sake or to satisfy my own curiosity or shame or my need to control or offer comfort?" We should pay attention to the process as well as the content, and frequently ask our clients versions of "What is it like for you to do this work with me? What can I do to make this process easier for you?"

In the above example, the social worker failed to engage with Ms. Echeverría empathically or to acknowledge the tremendous step she had taken in believing her daughter and asking Raúl to leave the family. The CPS worker was walking that delicate line between believing in a client and having faith in her, while at the same time trying to do her utmost to protect the child. The CPS worker might have had more success if she had conveyed more optimism to Ms. Echeverría and enlisted her involvement in a process of recovery, rather than shaming her for her daughter's abuse. Conveying hope about full recovery for the child, with clear steps to achieve that recovery, often encourages mothers both to cooperate with the services that are offered, and to devise healing attitudes and strategies of their own for their families.

## Avoiding Burnout and Improving Workplace Morale

The Springfield office of child protective services is a glum and depressing place to work. The staff seems overwhelmed by the severity of the conditions of the families in their caseload and with the lack of resources to help those families. There is a lot of turnover although some diehards have worked there for more than two decades. As their caseloads have grown and more work needs to be done on the computer, the employees interact with each other less. Much of the staff feels hopeless about helping their clients meaningfully, and the staff's hopelessness seems to feed into the clients' hopelessness, creating a pervading sense of gloom.

Working with children who have been victims of maltreatment and their families can be grim, indeed. It is difficult to face misery and cruelty on a daily basis, particularly when the victims are children. A long discussion of avoiding burnout is beyond the scope of this chapter. But I do want to include some mention of the importance of optimism because professionals who are burned out, tired of their work, and depressed are apt to experience greater difficulty in bonding with and enlisting the cooperation of clients who differ from them culturally.

For your sake and your clients' sake, I encourage you to take special note of those things that are going well. Small steps toward improved communication, signs of love, newfound assertiveness, the recovery of lost traditions—these can all be cause for celebration. At an agency where I worked we ended our group supervision meetings with a quick round of these "good news stories" (Fontes, 1995b). This helped change our demeanor as we left meetings. It also helped us stay attuned to signs of improvement and hope during the week, as we considered whether any particular observation, large or small, would be a "good one" to share during our "good news" story time.

I have worked with children's advocacy centers and CPS offices that were delightful and cheery. Although the employees heard stories similar to those of the CPS workers described previously, the supervisors were appreciative and worked hard to develop office morale. Employees felt appreciated. Employees were given an opportunity to decorate their work areas, and the agency provided a sense of belonging and support for innovative thinking. Of course, adequate salaries, time off, and other work benefits and conditions also help staff morale. The clients are served better when the staff is happier and more optimistic.

## Assessing Community Needs

When I first began to work in rural western Massachusetts, I was told that my ability to speak Spanish was of little interest to the agency because all the Latino clients were fluent in English. As soon as word of my presence at the agency got out, I was deluged by clients who spoke only Spanish.

Assess needs and you will find them. The Office of Minority Health (2001) recommends that agencies use census data, school enrollment data, and other sources of information to understand better the needs of their communities, and to plan the kinds of services needed. Most communities have a severe shortage of services to address the needs of immigrant, deaf, differently abled, cultural minority, and gay and lesbian clients. Contact community agencies and religious organizations and ask about the kinds of services they believe their constituents want and need.

It is also important to contact the consumers of our services directly. Once I worked with an agency that was trying to find a way to entice teen mothers into services. Finally, we asked the teenagers what *they* would like, and the teenagers replied that they would like to attend exercise classes that included baby-sitting services for their children. On the theory that the first step is an important one, the agency offered such services to the young women. Through the exercise classes, the women became less isolated, felt better about their bodies, and became more open to other kinds of services.

## Ensuring Multicultural Assessment, Consultation, and Training

> Although a children's advocacy center is located in a Haitian neighborhood, the center has never served a Haitian child or family. They brought in a consultant who offered a morning training on "working with diverse clients." One year later the agency still has not served a single Haitian child or family. The Haitian families are rarely involved with the child protection system, and when they are, the interviews are handled by child protective services without involving the children's advocacy center. Perhaps because of this, the child maltreatment cases involving Haitian families rarely go to court.

A cultural competency assessment is a "must" for every agency, and should be repeated at least once a decade to make sure the agency is working toward its goals and keeping up with changes in the community. A thorough assessment will help you identify strengths and problems, and promote action for improvement. (The Child Welfare League of America publishes several cultural competence assessment instruments.) Agencies often choose to bring in an outside consultant who can serve as a neutral party to assess the agency's current status in terms of cultural competency and begin to lay out a road map of where to go next. Unfortunately, some agencies wait until they are facing a discrimination suit by a former employee or client before engaging in this step.

Cultural competency is a journey that may begin with a general diversity training, but it should not stop there. Rather, agencies should engage their staff in increasingly sophisticated multicultural trainings (e.g., on antiracism, addressing the needs of specific ethnic populations or specific problems such as child sexual abuse, or in addressing the dynamics within the staff). If the trainings are of a high quality, they will not be superfluous or redundant.

Addressing issues of child maltreatment can be arduous. You may find yourself pulled in different directions by a variety of people with apparently conflicting goals: the family, the person who has been victimized, the person accused of offending, lawyers, protective workers, mental health personnel, police, and school staff. When the intervention is a cross-cultural encounter, these complexities increase dramatically. Supportive and knowledgeable supervision and consultation are absolute necessities. Issues of child maltreatment and culture are not easily handled with a seat-of-your-pants approach. We need to seek out opportunities to access new sources of information, including reading and attending workshops.

Agencies and teams that work with clients from a variety of ethnic groups often fail to plan adequately when they hire a "cultural consultant" to advise them in their work with specific cases or cultural groups (Stevenson & Renard, 1993). Some agencies hire a consultant to do a one-time workshop, and then assume that this has met the need for cultural competency training. However, as agency personnel become increasingly sophisticated about their work with multicultural issues, they will discover additional areas where they need to improve their knowledge and practice. Also, as new people come onto the staff, those people will need to be brought "up to speed" in terms of the agency's expectations for cultural competence.

The above are just some examples—earlier chapters of this book contain others—of what can go wrong when an agency fails to accommodate the needs of diverse clients and employees. In each case goodwill, hope, and an opportunity to make a difference are squandered, and the entire agency is impoverished because of a lack of cultural competency.

## CONCLUDING THOUGHTS

It is an exciting time for those of us who are working to improve the cultural competence of agencies and organizations in child maltreatment, and of the field itself. Changing demographics in the United States and Canada are requiring professionals to become skilled at meeting the needs of their diverse clients. At the same time, important government bodies and nongovernmental organizations are pushing their constituents to become more culturally competent. For example, the National Children's Alliance, which is the coordinating body of children's advocacy centers in the United States, considers cultural competency and diversity one of the 14 standards to be met by its centers. All the major professional bodies including the National Association of Social Workers, the American Psychological Association, the American Medical Association, and others include attention to cultural issues and competence in their code of ethics. A monocultural orientation is no longer an option.

The time is ripe for agencies to conduct the self-assessments and planning necessary to make sure they are offering the best services to clients from all cultural groups.

## QUESTIONS TO THINK ABOUT AND DISCUSS

1. Discuss where on the monocultural to multicultural spectrum you believe your agency (or college program) falls and why.

2. As an administrator (or if you were an administrator), what are three things you could do to improve the cultural competence of your child maltreatment agency?

3. What specific trainings would you like to see your agency undertake to improve its cultural competence in general and in regard to specific issues?

4. Imagine you are director of an agency in a community with a large Chinese immigrant population, and you currently have no Chinese-speaking staff members. Describe five steps that you would take to make sure your agency meets the needs of the Chinese people in your community.

# A Final Wish

I would like nothing more than to see this book become obsolete because child maltreatment has been eliminated, and because awareness of the needs of diverse cultural, racial, and economic groups has led to a more just society for all. I offer you my respect and thanks for taking every step you can to make sure all the children and families in your care receive the best possible professional response, which includes attending to cultural issues and eliminating bias in our systems.

# References

Abney, V. (2002). Cultural competency in the field of child maltreatment. In J. E. B. Myers, L. Berliner, J. Briere, C. Terry Hendrix, C. Jenny, & T. A. Reid (Eds.), *The APSAC handbook on child maltreatment* (2nd ed., pp. 477–486). Thousand Oaks, CA: Sage.

Abney, V. D., & Priest, R. (1995). African Americans and sexual child abuse. In L. A. Fontes (Ed.), *Sexual abuse in nine North American cultures: Treatment and prevention* (pp. 11–30). Newbury Park, CA: Sage.

Abujamra, A. (1995). A alma não tem cor [Recorded by Chico César]. *Aos vivos* [CD]. Sao Paulo: Velas.

Al-Hibri, A. Y. (1999). Is Western patriarchal feminism good for third world/minority women? In S. M. Okin, J.Cohen, M. Howard, & M. Nussbaum (Eds.), *Is multiculturalism bad for women?* (pp. 41–46). Princeton, NJ: Princeton University Press.

Almeida, R. V., & Dolan-Delvecchio, K. (1999). Addressing culture in batterers intervention: The Asian Indian community as an illustrative example. *Violence Against Women, 5*, 654–683.

Alvarez, J. (2004). *The woman I kept to myself.* Chapel Hill, NC: Algonquin Books.

American Academy of Pediatrics. (1998). Guidance for effective discipline. *Pediatrics, 101*, 723–728.

American Bar Association Commission on Domestic Violence. (2001, May). Teleconference, Civil Legal Assistance for Battered Immigrants.

American Professional Society on the Abuse of Children. (1995). *Practice guidelines: Use of anatomical dolls in child sexual abuse assessments.* Chicago: Author.

American Professional Society on the Abuse of Children. (2002). *Practice guidelines: Investigative interviewing in cases of alleged child abuse.* Chicago: Author.

Ards, S., Chung, C., & Myers, S. L. (1998). The effects of sample selection bias on racial differences in child abuse reporting. *Child Abuse and Neglect, 22*(2), 103–115.

Arey, D. (1995). Gay males and sexual child abuse. In L. A. Fontes (Ed.), *Sexual abuse in nine North American cultures: Treatment and prevention* (pp. 200–235). Newbury Park, CA: Sage.

Armstrong, L. (1995). *Of "sluts" and "bastards."* Monroe, ME: Common Courage Press.

Association of Chief Police Officers, Gender Working Group. (2000). *Dealing with cases of forced marriage.* London: Author.

Axtell, R. E. (1998). *Gestures: The do's and taboos of body language around the world* (rev. and exp. ed.). New York: Wiley.

Azzi-Lessing, L., & Olsen, L. (1996). Substance abuse-affected families in the child welfare system: New challenges, new alliances. *Social Work, 41*(1), 15–23.

Baird, C., Ereth, J., & Wagner, D. (1999). *Research-based risk assessment: Adding equity to CPS decision making.* Madison, WI: Children's Research Center, National Council on Crime and Delinquency.

Baker, K. A., & Dwairy, M. (2003). Cultural norms versus state law in treating incest: A suggested model for Arab families. *Child Abuse and Neglect, 27*(1), 109–123.

Baker, N. G. (1981). Social work through an interpreter. *Social Work, 26*, 391–397.

Bancroft, L., & Silverman, J. G. (2002). *The batterer as parent.* Thousand Oaks, CA: Sage.

Barnett, O. W., Martinez, T. E., & Keyson, M. (1996). The relationship between violence, social support, and self-blame in battered women. *Journal of Interpersonal Violence, 11*(2), 221–233.

Bass, E., & Davis, L. (2003). *Beginning to heal* (rev. ed.). New York: HarperCollins.

Beahl, L. E., Crouch, J. L., May, P. F., Valente, A. L., & Conyngham, H. A. (2001). Ethnicity in child maltreatment research: A content analysis. *Child Maltreatment, 6*, 143–147.

Belsky, J. (1980). Child maltreatment: An ecological integration. *American Psychologist, 35*, 320–335.

Borrego, J., Urquiza, A. J., Rasmussen, R. A., & Zebell, N. (1999). Parent–child interaction therapy with a family at high risk for physical abuse. *Child Maltreatment, 4*, 331–342.

Bottoms, B. L., & Shaver, P. R. (1995). In the name of God: A profile of religion-related child abuse. *Journal of Social Issues, 51*, 85–111.

Bowser, B. P., & Hunt, R. G. (Eds.). (1996). *Impacts of racism on white Americans* (2nd ed.). Thousand Oaks, CA: Sage.

Boyd-Franklin, N. (2003). *Black families in therapy* (2nd ed.): *Understanding the African American experience.* New York: Guilford Press.

Bradford, D. T., & Muñoz, A. (1993). Translation in bilingual psychotherapy. *Professional Psychology: Research and Practice, 24*, 52–61.

Bradley, C. R. (1998). Cultural interpretations of child discipline: Voices of African American scholars. *Family Journal, 6*, 272–278.

Bronfenbrenner, U. (1979). *The ecology of human development.* Cambridge, MA: Harvard University Press.

Burns, R. C., & Kaufman, S. H. (1972). *Actions, styles and symbols in kinetic family drawings: An interpretive manual.* New York: Brunner/Mazel.

Carnes, C. (2000). *Forensic evaluation of children when sexual abuse is suspected* (2nd ed.). Huntsville, AL: National Children's Advocacy Center.

Celano, M., Hazzard, A., Campbell, S. K., & Lang, C. B. (2002). Attribution retraining with sexually abused children: Review of techniques. *Child Maltreatment, 7,* 65–76.

Chan, C. S. (1999). Culture, sexuality, and shame: A Korean American woman's experience. In Y. M. Jenkins (Ed.), *Diversity in college settings: Directives for helping professionals* (pp. 77–85). New York: Routledge.

Chan, S. (1992). Families with Asian roots. In E. W. Lynch & M. J. Hanson (Eds.), *Developing cross-cultural competence: A guide for working with young children and their families* (pp. 181–257). Baltimore: Brookes.

Charlow, A. (2001–2002). Race, poverty and neglect. *William Mitchell Law Review, 28,* 763–790.

Chesapeake Institute. (1993). *Investigative interviewing techniques in child sexual abuse cases* [Videotape]. Thousand Oaks, CA: Sage.

Children's Research Center (2003). Risk assessment in child welfare. Retrieved August 5, 2003, from *http://www.nccd-crc.org/crcindex.htm*

Chipungu, S. S., & Bent-Goodley, T. B. (2003). Race, poverty and child maltreatment. *APSAC Advisor, 15*(2), 9–10.

Collier, A. F., McClure, F. H., Collier, J., Otto, C., & Polloi, A. (1999). Culture-specific views of child maltreatment and parenting styles in a Pacific-Island community. *Child Abuse and Neglect, 23,* 229–244.

Cooper, L. A., & Powe, N. R (2004). *Disparities in patient experiences, health care processes, and outcomes: The role of patient–provider racial, ethnic, and language concordance.* New York: Commonwealth Fund.

Coulton, C. J., Korbin, J. E., & Su, M. (1999). Neighborhoods and child maltreatment: A multilevel study. *Child Abuse and Neglect, 23,* 1019–1040.

Crago, M. B. (1992). Communicative interaction and second language acquisition: An Inuit example. *TESOL Quarterly, 26,* 487–505.

Crouch, J. L., & Behl, L. E. (2001). Relationships among parental beliefs in corporal punishment, reported stress, and physical child abuse potential. *Child Abuse and Neglect, 25,* 413–419.

Cyr, M., Wright, J., McDuff, P., & Perron, A. (2002). Intrafamilial sexual abuse: Brother–sister incest does not differ from father–daughter and stepfather–stepdaughter incest. *Child Abuse and Neglect, 26,* 957–973.

Danticat, E. (1994). *Breath, eyes, memory.* New York: Random House.

Daro, D. (1994). Prevention of child sexual abuse. *The Future of Children, 4*(2), 198–223.

Daro, D. (2003). Child abuse prevention: Accomplishments and challenges. *APSAC Advisor, 15*(2), 3–4.

Daro, D., & Cohn Donnelly, A. (2002). Child abuse prevention: Accomplishments and challenges. In J. Myers, L. Berliner, J. Briere, C. T. Hendrix, C. Jenny, & T. A. Reid (Eds.), *The APSAC handbook on child maltreatment* (2nd ed., pp. 431–448). Thousand Oaks, CA: Sage.

Daro, D., & Gelles, R. J. (1992). Public attitudes and behaviors with respect to child abuse prevention. *Journal of Interpersonal Violence, 7,* 517–531.

Davidson, B. (2000). The interpreter as institutional gatekeeper: The social–linguistic role of interpreters in Spanish–English medical discourse. *Journal of Sociolinguistics, 4,* 379–405.

Davis, P. W. (1999). Corporal punishment cessation: Social contexts and parents' experiences. *Journal of Interpersonal Violence, 14,* 492–510.

Davis, S. L., & Bottoms, B. L. (2002). Effects of social support on children's eye-witness reports: A test of the underlying mechanism. *Law and Human Behavior, 26,* 185–215.

DeBruyn, L., Chino, M., Serna, P., & Fullerton-Gleason, L. (2001). Child maltreatment in American Indian and Alaska Native communities: Integrating culture, history, and public health for intervention and prevention. *Child Maltreatment, 6,* 89–102.

De La Cruz-Quiroz, G. (2000, June). *Working with Latino families on issues of child sexual abuse.* Paper presented at the American Professional Society on the Abuse of Children Colloquium, Chicago, IL.

Delpit, L. (2002). No kinda sense. In L. Delpit & J. K. Dowdy (Eds.), *The skin that we speak* (pp. 31–48). New York: New Press.

Delson, N., Gaba, R. J., & Walker, J. (2003). *Family violence response teams: Building community capacity to prevent family violence.* Davis: University of California, Davis, Center for Human Services.

DeYoung, Y., & Zigler, E. F. (1994). Machismo in two cultures: Relation to punitive child-rearing practices. *American Journal of Orthopsychiatry, 64,* 386–395.

Dowdy, J. K. (2002). Ovuh dyuh. In L. Delpit & J. K. Dowdy (Eds.), *The skin that we speak* (pp. 3–13). New York: New Press.

Dubowitz, H. (1999). *Neglected children: Research, practice and policy.* Newbury Park, CA: Sage

Dunkerley, G. K., & Dalenberg, C. J. (1999). Secret-keeping behaviors in black and white children as a function of interviewer race, racial identity, and risk for abuse. *Journal of Aggression, Maltreatment and Trauma, 2,* 13–35.

Duong, I. (2003). *Traditional medicine and child abuse.* Workshop presented at the American Professional Society on the Abuse of Children Colloquium, Orlando, FL.

Durrant, J. E., Ensom, R., & the Coalition on Physical Punishment of Children and Youth. (2004). *Joint statement on physical punishment of children and youth.* Ottawa: Children's Hospital of Eastern Ohio.

Edleson, J. L. (1999). The overlap between woman abuse and child abuse. *Violence Against Women, 5,* 134–154.

Elliott, A. N., & Carnes, C. N. (2001). Reactions of nonoffending parents to the sexual abuse of their children: A review of the literature. *Child Maltreatment, 6,* 314–331.

Emory University. (1999). Dictionary of socio-rhetorical terms. Retrieved June 17, 2003, from *http://www.emory.edu/COLLEGE/RELIGION/faculty/robbins/SRI/defns/h_defns.html*

Eron, L. D. (1996). Research and public policy. *Pediatrics, 98,* 821–823.

Erzinger, S. (1999). Communication between Spanish-speaking patients and their doctors in medical encounters. In G. X. Ma & G. Henderson (Eds.), *Rethinking ethnicity and health care: A sociocultural perspective* (pp. 122–140). Springfield, IL: C. C. Thomas.

Faber, A., & Mazlich, E. (1991). *Cómo hablar para que los niños escuchen y cómo escuchar para que los niños hablen.* Mexico City, Mexico: Edivision.

Fadiman, A. (1997). *The spirit catches you and you fall down.* New York: Farrar, Straus & Giroux.

Falicov, C. J. (1995). Training to think culturally: A multidimensional comparative framework. *Family Process, 34,* 373–88.

Falicov, C. J. (1996). Mexican families. In M. McGoldrick, J. Giordano, & J. K. Pearce (Eds.), *Ethnicity and family therapy* (2nd ed., pp. 169–182). New York: Guilford Press.

Falicov, C. J. (1998). *Latino families in therapy.* New York: Guilford Press.

Faller, K. (1999). Focused questions for interviewing children suspected of maltreatment and other traumatic experiences. *APSAC Advisor, 12*(1), 14–18.

Federal Interagency Forum on Child and Family Statistics. (2004). America's children in brief: Key national indicators of well-being, 2004. Retrieved September 14, 2004, from *http://www.childstats.gov/ac2004/intro.asp*

Feiring, C., Taska, L., & Lewis, M. (2002). Adjustment following sexual abuse discovery: The role of shame and attributional style. *Developmental Psychology, 38,* 79–92.

Ferrari, A. M. (2002). The impact of culture upon child rearing practices and definitions of maltreatment. *Child Abuse and Neglect, 26,* 793–813.

Finkelhor, D., Asdigian, N., & Dzuba-Leatherman, J. (1993, August). *Victimization prevention training in action: A national survey of children's experiences coping with actual threats and assaults.* Durham, NH: University of New Hampshire, Family Research Laboratory.

Finkelhor, D., & Korbin, J. (1988). Child abuse as an international issue. *Child Abuse and Neglect, 12,* 3–23.

Firestone, D. (2001, March 30). Child abuse at a church creates a stir in Atlanta. *New York Times,* p. A14.

Fitzpatrick, K. M., & Boldizar, J. (1993). The prevalence and consequences of exposure to violence among African-American youth. *Journal of the American Academy of Child and Adolescent Psychiatry, 32,* 424–430.

Fontes, L. A. (1993a). Considering culture and oppression: Steps toward an ecology of sexual child abuse. *Journal of Feminist Family Therapy, 5*(1), 25–54.

Fontes, L. A. (1993b). Disclosures of sexual abuse by Puerto Rican children: Oppression and cultural barriers. *Journal of Child Sexual Abuse, 2*(1), 21–35.

Fontes, L. A. (Ed.). (1995a). *Sexual abuse in nine North American cultures: Treatment and prevention.* Newbury Park, CA: Sage.

Fontes, L. A. (1995b). Sharevision: Collaborative supervision and self-care strategies for working with trauma. *Family Journal, 3,* 249–254.

Fontes, L. A. (1997). Conducting ethical cross-cultural research on family violence. In G. K. Kantor & J. L. Jasinski (Eds.), *Out of the darkness: Contemporary research perspectives on family violence* (pp. 296–312).

Fontes, L. A. (2000). Working with Latino families on issues of child abuse and ne-
    glect. *National Child Advocate, 3*(2), 1, 4–7.
Fontes, L. A. (Ed.). (2001). Cultural issues in child maltreatment [Special Issue].
    *Child Maltreatment, 6.*
Fontes, L. A. (2002). Child discipline and physical abuse in immigrant Latino fami-
    lies: Reducing violence and misunderstanding. *Journal of Counseling and De-
    velopment, 80,* 31–40.
Fontes, L. A., Cruz, M., & Tabachnick, J. (2001). Views of child sexual abuse in
    two cultural communities: An exploratory study among African Americans
    and Latinos. *Child Maltreatment, 6,* 103–117.
Freed, A. O. (1988). Interviewing through an interpreter. *Social Work, 33,* 315–318.
Friedrich, W. N. (1990). Group therapy with child and adolescent victims. In *Psy-
    chotherapy with sexually abused boys* (pp. 210–226). New York: Norton.
Friedrich, W. N. (1995). *Psychotherapy with sexually abused boys.* Thousand
    Oaks, CA: Sage.
Friedrich, W. N., Grambsch, P., Damon, L., Hewitt, S., Koverola, C., Lang, R.,
    Wolfe, V., & Broughton, D. (1992). The Child Sexual Behavior Inventory:
    Normative and clinical contrasts. *Psychological Assessment, 4,* 303–311.
García, C. (1992). *Dreaming in Cuban.* New York: Ballantine.
García Coll, C. T. (1990). Developmental outcome of minority infants: A process
    oriented look at our beginnings. *Child Development, 61,* 270–289.
Gardner, R. A. (1973). *The talking, feeling, and doing game.* Cresskill, NJ:
    Creative Therapeutics.
Gentile, D. A., & Walsh, D. A. (2002). A normative study of family media habits.
    *Applied Developmental Psychology, 23,* 157–178.
Gibson, L. E., & Leitenberg, H. (2000). Child sexual abuse prevention programs:
    Do they decrease the occurrence of child sexual abuse? *Child Abuse and
    Neglect, 24*(9), 1115–1125.
Gil, E. (1988). *Outgrowing the pain.* New York: Dell.
Gil, E. (1996a). *Systemic treatment of families who abuse.* San Francisco: Jossey-Bass.
Gil, E. (1996b). *Treating abused adolescents.* New York: Guilford Press.
Giles-Sims, J., Straus, M. A., & Sugarman, D. B. (1995). Child, maternal and fam-
    ily characteristics associated with spanking. *Family Relations, 44,* 170–176.
Gomez, M. (2004). *AmaXonica: Howls from the left side of my body* [CD].
    Longmeadow, MA: Rotary Records.
Grauerholz, L. (2000). An ecological approach to understanding sexual revictimiz-
    ation: Linking personal, interpersonal, and sociocultural factors and pro-
    cesses. *Child Maltreatment, 5,* 5–17.
Graziano, A. M. (1994). Why we should study subabusive violence against chil-
    dren. *Journal of Interpersonal Violence, 9,* 412–419.
Hahm, H. C., & Guterman, N. B. (2001). The emerging problem of physical child
    abuse in South Korea. *Child Maltreatment, 6,* 169–179.
Hamburg, D. (1992). *Today's children: Creating a future for a generation in crisis.*
    New York: Times Books.
Hardy, M. (1998). Ten tips on using court interpreters in child witness cases. *Na-
    tional Center for Prosecution of Child Abuse, Update, 11*(12), 1–2.

Hassan, R. (2004, April). *Identifying child abuse across cultures: Somali families.* Paper presented at Baystate Health Systems Conference, Springfield, MA.

Hauck, F. R., Herman, S. M., Donovan, M., Iyasu, S., Merrick Moore, C. A., Donoghue, E. R., Kirschner, R. H., & Willinger, M. (2003). Sleep environment and the risk of sudden infant death syndrome in an urban population: The Chicago infant mortality study. *Pediatrics, 111,* 1207–1214.

Herman, J. L. (1981). *Father–daughter incest.* Cambridge, MA: Harvard University Press.

Hines, P. M., & Boyd-Franklin, N. (1996). African American families. In M. McGoldrick, J. Giordano, & J. K. Pearce (Eds.), *Ethnicity and family therapy* (2nd ed., pp. 66–84). New York: Guilford Press.

Holmes, L. S., & Vieth, V. I. (2003). Finding words/half a nation: The forensic interview training program of CornerHouse and APRI's national center for prosecution of child abuse. *APSAC Advisor, 15*(1), 4–8.

Holton, J. K. (1993). Preventing child sexual abuse in the African American community without reinventing the wheel. *APSAC Advisor, 6*(1), 25.

Holzman, C. (1995). Rethinking the role of guilt and shame in white women's antiracism work. In J. Adleman & G. Enguídanos (Eds.), *Racism in the lives of women* (pp. 325–332). New York: Harrington Park Press.

Howard, B. J. (1996). Advising parents on discipline: What works. *Pediatrics, 98,* 809–815.

Ide, K. (1995). Not telling stories: A Japanese way. *Family Journal, 3,* 259–264.

Ima, K., & Hohm, C. (1991). Child maltreatment among Asian and Pacific Islander refugees and immigrants. *Journal of Interpersonal Violence, 6,* 267–285.

Javed, N. S. (1995). Salience of loss and marginality: Life themes of "immigrant women of color" in Canada. In J. Adleman & G. Enguídanos (Eds.), *Racism in the lives of women* (pp. 13–22). New York: Harrington Park Press.

Jenny, C. (2002). Medical issues in child sexual abuse. In J. Myers, L. Berliner, T. Briere, C. T. Hendrix, C. Jenny, & T. A. Reid (Eds.), *The APSAC handbook on child maltreatment* (2nd ed., pp. 235–247). Thousand Oaks, CA: Sage.

Joe, J. R., & Malach, R. S. (1994). Families with Native American roots. In E. W. Lynch & M. J. Hanson (Eds.), *Developing cross-cultural competence: A guide for working with young children and their families* (pp. 89–115). Baltimore: Brookes.

Johnson, K. K. (1998). Crime or punishment: The parental corporal punishment defense—reasonable and necessary, or excused abuse? *University of Illinois Law Review,* 413–487.

Johnson, T. C. (1999). *Understanding your child's sexual behavior.* Oakland, CA: New Harbinger.

Jones, L. M., Finkelhor, D., & Kopiec, K. (2001). Why is sexual abuse declining? A survey of state child protection administrators. *Child Abuse and Neglect, 25,* 1139–1158.

Kamerman, S. B., & Kahn, A. J. (1993). Home health visiting in Europe. *Future of Children, 3*(3), 39–52.

Kamerman, S. B., & Kahn, A. J. (1990). The problems facing social services for children, youth, and families. *Children and Youth Services Review, 12*(1/2), 1–184.

Kapp, S. A., McDonald, T. P., & Diamond, K. L (2001). The path to adoption for children of color. *Child Abuse and Neglect, 25,* 215–229.

Kim, H. S., & Markus, H. R. (2002). Freedom of speech and freedom of silence: An analysis of talking as cultural practice. In R. A. Shweder, M. Minow, & H. R. Markus (Eds.), *Engaging cultural differences: The multicultural challenge in liberal democracies* (pp. 432–452). New York: Russell Sage Foundation.

Kingsolver, B. (1995). *High tide in Tucson.* New York: HarperCollins.

Klass, P. (2004, August 31). Month by month, a tiny baby's hard-won pounds. *New York Times,* pp. D5, D8.

Kohl, H. (2002). Topsy-turvies: Teacher talk and student talk. In L. Delpit & J. K. Dowdy (Eds.), *The skin that we speak* (pp. 145–161). New York: New Press.

Kolko, D. (1996). Individual cognitive behavioral treatment and family therapy for physically abused children and their offending parents: A comparison of clinical outcomes. *Child Maltreatment, 1,* 322–342.

Kolko, D. J., & Feiring, C. (Eds.). (2002). Special focus section on children's attribututions about abuse. *Child Maltreatment, 7.*

Korbin, J. E., & Spilsbury, J. C. (1999). Cultural competence and child neglect. In H. Dubowitz (Ed.), *Neglected children: Research, practice and policy* (pp. 69–88). Newbury Park, CA: Sage.

Krajewski-Jaime, E. R. (1991). Folk-healing among Mexican-American families as a consideration in the delivery of child welfare and child health care services. *Child Welfare, 70,* 157–167.

Lahiri, J. (1999). *Interpreter of maladies.* Boston: Houghton Mifflin.

Lambert, W. (2002, June). *Corporal punishment: How much is too much?* Paper presented at the American Professional Society on the Abuse of Children Colloquium, New Orleans, LA.

Levesque, R. J. R. (2001). *Culture and family violence: Fostering change through human rights law.* Washington, DC: American Psychological Association.

Lewis, A. D. (Ed.). (1999). *Cultural diversity in sexual abuser treatment.* Brandon, VT: Safer Society Press.

Ligezinska, M., Firestone, P., Manion, I. G., McIntyre, J., Ensom, R., & Wells, G. (1996). Children's emotional and behavioral reactions following the disclosure of extrafamilial sexual abuse: Initial effects. *Child Abuse and Neglect, 20*(2), 111–125.

Lipson, J. G. (1993). Ethics and intervention in ethnography. In J. Morse (Ed.), *Critical issues in qualitative research* (pp. 333–355). Newbury Park, CA: Sage.

Lipson, J. G., Dibble, S. L., & Minarik, P. A. (1996). *Culture and nursing care: A pocket guide.* San Francisco: University of California, San Francisco, School of Nursing.

Lockhart, L. L. (1985). Methodological issues in comparative racial analyses: The case of wife abuse. *Social Work Research and Abstracts, 21,* 35–41.

Magana, J. R. (1991). Sex, drugs, and HIV: An ethnographic approach. *Social Science and Medicine, 32*(1), 5–9.

Maiter, S. (2003). The context of culture: Social work practice with Canadians of South Asian background. In A. Al-Krenawi & J. R. Graham (Eds.), *Multicultural social work in Canada* (pp. 365–387). New York: Oxford University Press.

Maiter, S., Alaggia, R., & Trocmé, N. (2004). Perceptions of child maltreatment by parents from the Indian subcontinent: Challenging myths about culturally based abusive parenting practices. *Child Maltreatment, 9,* 309–324.

Maiter, S., Trocmé, N., & Shakir, U. (1999). Fabricating tools of resistance. In *Qualitative analysis conference: The interdisciplinary study of social process,* St. Thomas University, New Brunswick, Canada.

Marneffe, C. (1996). Child abuse treatment: A fallow land. *Child Abuse and Neglect, 20,* 379–384.

Martínez, R. (2003, July 23). *Santería and Afro-Cuban religions and child abuse.* Workshop presented at the American Professional Society on the Abuse of Children annual colloquium, Orlando, FL.

McCord, J. (1996). Unintended consequences of punishment. *Pediatrics, 98,* 832–834.

McDonald, E. (2004). *Adolescent pregnancy prevention from the perspectives of adolescent mothers and national policymakers: An interpretive policy analysis.* Unpublished doctoral dissertation, Brandeis University, Waltham, MA.

McIntosh, P. (1998). White privilege: Unpacking the invisible knapsack. In M. McGoldrick (Ed.), *Revisioning family therapy: Race, culture, and gender in clinical practice* (pp. 147–152). New York: Guilford Press.

Mederos, F. (2003, June 2). Comments to share (from Fernando Mederos). Message posted to *http://mapnp.mnforum.org/pipermail.pemv-net/2003/000171.html*

Melton, G. B. (2003, October). *Mandated reporting: A policy without reason.* Commentary prepared for a virtual discussion sponsored by the International Society for Prevention of Child Abuse and Neglect.

Minarik, P. A. (1996). Diversity among spiritual and religious beliefs. In J. G. Lipson, S. L. Dibble, & P. A. Minarik (Eds.), *Culture and nursing care: A pocket guide* (pp. B1–B21). San Francisco: University of California, San Francisco, School of Nursing.

Morsbach, H. (1988). The importance of silence and stillness in Japanese nonverbal communication: A cross-cultural approach. In F. Poyatos (Ed.), *Cross-cultural perspectives in nonverbal communication* (pp. 201–215). Lewiston, NY: Hogrefe.

Mosby, L., Rawls, A. W., Meehan, A. J., Mays, E., & Pettinari, C. J. (1999). Troubles in interracial talk about discipline: An examination of African American childrearing narratives. *Journal of Comparative Family Studies, 30,* 489–521.

Myers, S. L. (2003). Why are children of color overrepresented in reports to child protective services? *APSAC Advisor, 15*(2), 10–11.

Negroni, L. (1998). *Puerto Rican mothers' thoughts and attitudes about child discipline and child abuse: Their attributions and expectations of children.* Unpublished doctoral dissertation, Boston College, Boston, MA.

New South Wales Environmental Protection Agency. (2004). Traditional remedies reported to contain lead. Retrieved August 25, 2004, from *http://www.epa.nsw.gov.au/leadsafe/remedies.htm*

Okamura, A., Heras, P., & Wong-Kerberg, L. (1995). Asian, Pacific Island, and Filipino Americans and child sexual abuse. In L. Fontes (Ed.), *Sexual abuse in nine North American cultures: Treatment and prevention* (pp. 67–96). Newbury Park, CA: Sage.

Okin, S. M. (1999). *Is multiculturalism bad for women?* Princeton, NJ: Princeton University Press.

Orenstein, D. (1994). *Lifecycles: Jewish women on life passages and personal milestones.* Woodstock, VT: Jewish Lights.

Payne, M. A. (1989). Use and abuse of corporal punishment: A Caribbean view. *Child Abuse and Neglect, 13,* 389–401.

Pearce, J. W., & Pezzot-Pearce, T. D. (1997). *Psychotherapy of abused and neglected children.* New York: Guilford Press.

Plummer, C. A. (2001). Prevention of child sexual abuse: A survey of 87 programs. *Violence and Victims, 16*(5), 575–588.

Plummer, C. A. (2004). Prevention is appropriate, prevention is successful. In R. Gelles & D. Loseke (Eds.), *Current controversies on family violence* (2nd ed., pp. 288–305). Newbury Park, CA: Sage.

Popkin, M. H. (1998). *1–2–3–4 Padres* (Parenting curriculum, leader's guide, and video in Spanish). Atlanta, GA: Active Parenting.

Purcell-Gates, V. (2002). ". . . As soon as she opened her mouth!": Issues of language, literacy, and power. In L. Delpit & J. K. Dowdy (Eds.), *The skin that we speak* (pp. 121–141). New York: New Press.

Qureshi, B. (1989). Multicultural aspects of child abuse in Britain. *Journal of the Royal Society of Medicine, 82,* 65–66.

Reed, L. D. (1993). Enhancing children's resistance to misleading questions during forensic interviews. *APSAC Advisor, 6*(2), 3–8.

Roberts, D. (2002). *Shattered bonds: The color of child welfare.* New York: Basic Books.

Rogoff, B. (2003). *The cultural nature of human development.* New York: Oxford University Press.

Roland, A. (1994). Identity, self, and individualism in a multicultural perspective. In E. P. Salett & D. R. Koslow (Eds.), *Race, ethnicity, and self* (pp. 11–23). Washington, DC: National MultiCultural Institute.

Rose, G. (1992). *The strategy of preventive medicine.* Oxford, UK: Oxford University Press.

Ross, S. M. (1996). Risk of physical abuse to children of spouse abusing parents. *Child Abuse and Neglect, 20,* 589–598.

Rosser, B. S., Coleman, E., & Ohmans, P. (1993). Safer sex maintenance and reduction of unsafe sex among homosexually active men: A new therapeutic approach. *Health Education Research, 8,* 19–34.

Rounds, K. A. (1986). Responding to AIDS: Rural community strategies. *Social Casework, 69*(6), 360–365.

Russell, D. E. H. (1986). *The secret traume: Incest in the lives of girls and women.* New York: Basic Books.

Saba, G. W., & Rodgers, D. V. (1990). Discrimination in urban family practice: Lessons from poor minority families. In G. W. Saba, B. M. Karrer, & K. V. Hardy (Eds.), *Minorities and family therapy* (pp. 177–207). New York: Haworth.

Sapphire. (1996). *Push*. New York: Random House.

Schilling, R., Schinke, S., Nichols, S., Zayas, L., Miller, S., Orlandi, M., & Botvin, G. (1989). Developing strategies for AIDS prevention research with black and Hispanic drug users. *Public Health Reports, 104*(1), 2–11.

Scully, M., Kuoch, T., & Miller, R. A. (1995). Cambodians and child sexual abuse. In L. A. Fontes (Ed.), *Sexual abuse in nine North American cultures: Treatment and prevention* (pp. 97–127). Newbury Park, CA: Sage.

Sedlak, A. J., Bruce, C., & Schultz, D. J. (2001). Letter to the editor. *Child Abuse and Neglect, 25*, 1–5.

Shipman, K. L., Rossman, B. B. R., & West, J. C. (1999). Co-occurrence of spousal violence and child abuse: Conceptual implications. *Child Maltreatment, 4*, 93–102.

Showers, J., & Bandman, R. L. (1986). Scarring for life: Abuse with electric cords. *Child Abuse and Neglect, 10*, 25–31.

Smith, E. (2002). Ebonics: A case history. In L. Delpit & J. K. Dowdy (Eds.), *The skin that we speak* (pp. 15–30). New York: New Press.

Socolar, R. R. S., & Runyan, D. K. (2001). Unusual manifestations of child abuse. In R. M. Reece & S. Ludwig (Eds.), *Child abuse: Medical diagnosis and management* (pp. 453–466). Hagerstown, MD: Lippincott Williams & Wilkins.

Steele, K. (1989). Sitting with the shattered soul. *Pilgrimage, 15*(6), 19–25.

Stevenson, H. C., & Renard, G. (1993). Trusting ol' wise owls: Therapeutic use of cultural strengths in African American families. *Professional Psychology: Research and Practice, 24*, 433–442.

Stewart, C. L., Lara, M. G., Amighetti, L. D. H., Wissow, L. S., Guitierrez, M. I., Levav, I., & Maddaleno, M. (2000). Parenting and physical punishment: Primary care interventions in Latin America. *Pan American Journal of Public Health, 8*, 257–267.

Stone, R. (2004). *No secrets no lies: How Black families can heal from sexual abuse*. New York: Broadway Books.

Strassberg, Z., Dodge, K. A., Pettit, G. S., & Bates, J. E. (1994). Spanking in the home and children's subsequent aggression toward kindergarten peers. *Development and Psychopathology, 6*, 445–461.

Straus, M. A., & Donnelly, D. A. (2001). *Beating the devil out of them: Corporal punishment in American families and its effect on children* (2nd ed.). New York: Lexington Books.

Straus, M. A., & Lauer, S. (1992). *Corporal punishment of children and crime in ethnic group context*. Paper presented the American Society of Criminology conference, New Orleans, LA. (Available from the Family Research Laboratory, Durham, NH, 03824)

Straus, M. A., & Mathur, A. K. (1994). *Corporal punishment by parents and later occupational and economic achievement of children*. Durham, NH: Family Research Laboratory.

Straus, M. A., & Mathur, A. K. (1996). Social change and the trends in approval of corporal punishment by parents from 1968–1994. In D. Frehsee, W. Horn, & K. D. Bussmann (Eds.), *Family violence against children: A challenge for society* (pp. 91–105). New York: Walter de Gruyter.

Sue, D. W., & Sue, D. (2003). *Counseling the culturally diverse* (4th ed.). New York: Wiley.

Sutherland, A. (1996). Gypsies (Roma). In J. G. Lipson, S. L. Dibble, & P. A. Minarik (Eds.), *Culture and nursing care: A pocket guide* (pp. 126–138). San Francisco: University of California, San Francisco, School of Nursing.

Swan, R. (1998). Religion-based medical neglect and corporal punishment must not be tolerated. *APSAC Advisor, 11*(1), 2–3.

Taylor, C., & Fontes, L. A. (1995). Seventh Day Adventists and sexual child abuse. In L. A. Fontes (Ed.), *Sexual abuse in nine North American cultures: Treatment and prevention* (pp. 176–199). Newbury Park, CA: Sage.

Terao, S. Y., Borrego, J. J., & Urquiza, A. J. (2001). A reporting and response model to culture and child maltreatment. *Child Maltreatment, 6,* 158–168.

Texas Department of State Health Services. (2004). Childhood lead poisoning prevention. Retrieved September 2004 from *http://www.r03.tdh.state.tx.us/LeadScreening.htm*

Thomas, J. N. (1998, July 8). *School-based prevention: Strategies for working with African-American children.* Paper presented at the American Professional Society on the Abuse of Children 6th National Colloquium, Chicago, IL.

Tjaden, P. G., & Thoennes, N. (1992). Predictors of legal intervention in child maltreatment cases. *Child Abuse and Neglect, 16,* 807–821.

Tobin, P., & Kessner, S. L. (2002). *Keeping kids safe: Child sexual abuse prevention manual.* Alameda, CA: Hunter House.

Trepper, T. S., & Barrett, M. J. (1989). *Systemic treatment of incest: A therapeutic handbook.* New York: Brunner/Mazel.

U.S. Department of Health and Human Services, Administration for Children and Families. (2002). *Child maltreatment 2002.* Washington, DC: Author.

U.S. Department of Health and Human Services, Administration for Children and Families. (2003). Emerging practices in the prevention of child abuse and neglect. Retrieved July 2, 2003, from *http://www.calib.com/nccanch/prevention/emerging/report/maltreatment.cfm#one*

U.S. Department of Health and Human Services, National Center on Child Abuse and Neglect. (1996). *National incidence study* (NIS-3). Washington, DC: Author.

U.S. Department of Health and Human Services, Office of Civil Rights. (1998). *Guidance memorandum on prohibition against national origin discrimination: Persons with limited English proficiency.* Washington, DC: Author.

U.S. Department of Health and Human Services, Office of Minority Health. (2001). *National standards for culturally and linguistically appropriate services in health care.* Rockville, MD: IQ Solutions.

U.S. Department of State. (2004, June 14). *Trafficking in persons report* (International Information Programs). Washington, DC: Author.

Vanderhorst, K. R. (1996). *Rearing African children under American occupation.* Washington, DC: Hotep Productions.

Wilson, M. (1994). *Crossing the boundary: Black women survive incest.* Seattle: Seal Press.

Woldeguiorguis, I. M. (2003). Racism and sexism in child welfare. Effects on women of color as mothers and practitioners. *Child Welfare, 84,* 273–288.

World Health Organization. (1998). *Care of the umbilical cord: A review of the evidence*. Geneva, Switzerland: Author.

Yang, J. A. (2004). Marriage by capture in the Hmong culture: The legal issue of cultural rights versus women's rights. *Law and Society Review at UCSB, 3*, 38–49.

Yep, G. (1994). HIV/AIDS education and prevention for Asian and Pacific Islander communities: Toward the development of general guidelines. *AIDS Education and Prevention, 6*(2), 184–186.

Youssef, R. M., Attia, M. S., & Kamel, M. I. (1998). Children experiencing violence, I: Parental use of corporal punishment. *Child Abuse and Neglect, 22*, 959–973.

Yuksel, S. (2000). Collusion and denial of childhood sexual trauma in traditional societies. In A. Y. Shalev, R. Yehuda, & A. C. McFarlane (Eds.), *International handbook of human response to trauma* (pp. 153–162). New York: Kluwer.

Zayas, L. H. (1992). Childrearing, social stress, and child abuse: Clinical considerations with Hispanic families. *Journal of Social Distress and the Homeless, 1*, 291–309.

Zayas, L. H., & Solari, F. (1994). Early childhood socialization in Hispanic families: Context, culture, and practice implications. *Professional Psychology: Research and Practice, 25*, 200–206.

Zellman, G. L., & Fair, C. C. (2002). Preventing and reporting abuse. In J. Myers, L. Berliner, J. Briere, C. T. Hendrix, C. Jenny, & T. A. Reid (Eds.), *The APSAC handbook on child maltreatment* (2nd ed., pp. 449–475). Thousand Oaks, CA: Sage.

Zuravin, S. J. (1989). The ecology of child abuse and neglect: Review of the literature and presentation of data. *Violence and Victims, 4*, 101–129.

# Index

Quality of services, 204–205
Questioning
  about sexual abuse, 138–139
  to gather information, 94–95

Race
  definition of, 5–6
  disproportionality of in child welfare
    system, 10, 61, 81, 177
  social class and, 111
Racial harassment, 205–206
Racism, 6, 14, 112, 124, 155, 194, 211
Rape and forced marriage, 44, 45
Rapport, building, 89, 90–92
Recruitment
  of bilingual staff, 205
  of diverse staff, 206–208
Refugee, definition of, 47
Refugee status and truthfulness, 49, 50,
  51
Religion and corporal punishment, 113–
  114, 118. *See also* Catholic religion;
  Jewish religion; Muslim religion;
  Sikh religion
Reporting suspicions of child abuse
  cultural issues and, 60–63
  in presence of caretaker, 121
  racial and economic bias in, 26, 61, 62
Resistance, 6
Resources
  for families, accessing, 25
  sharing among family members, 66
Respect, conveying, 25, 52, 197–198
Responsibility for sexual abuse,
  assignment of, 139–142, 144–145
Revictimization, 153–154
Ringworm, 10
Rituals or ceremonies
  cleansing, 146
  shame-releasing, 157
Roberts, D., 10, 26, 60, 61, 70
Rogoff, B., 3, 9, 38, 65, 77
Russell, D. E. H., 153

Schools
  academic success and corporal
    punishment, 127–128
  child sexual abuse prevention
    programs in, 183–184
  immigrant families and, 39–41

Seating arrangements for interviews,
  103–104
Secondary prevention programming,
  179–180
Sexual abuse. *See also* Shame
  anger at perpetrator of, 142–143
  cultural justifications for, 79
  damaged goods concept and, 145–146
  individual response to, 136
  interviewing clients about, 138–139
  prevention of, 182–184
  responsibility for, assignment of, 139–
    142, 144–145
  sexual play or acting out following,
    151–152, 153
Sexuality education, 140, 146
Sexual matters, discussing, 92–93
Shame
  centrality of in sexual abuse, 135
  counteracting, 156–158
  culture and, 138
  damaged goods concept and, 145–146
  definition of, 135
  failure to protect and, 142–143
  fate and, 143–145
  layers of, 154–156
  predictions of shameful future, 150–
    153
  responsibility for sexual abuse and,
    139–142, 144–145
  revictimization and, 153–154
  sexual abuse and, 136–139
  virginity and, 146–150
Shaping interventions, 3–4
Sharing resources, 66
Sickle-cell anemia, 10
SIDS (sudden infant death syndrome),
  65
Sikh religion, 72
Silence in interview, 105–106
Simultaneous interpreting, 172–173
Size of child, 67
Slavery, history of, 118, 127
Slave trade in immigrants, 40
Slavic cultures, 24
Sleeping arrangements, 64–65
Social class
  ethnic issues compared to, 14
  filing report and, 61
  language and, 17
  poverty and, 18–19